the
simple, healing cleanse

WITH MORE THAN 50 WHOLE FOOD RECIPES

the
simple, healing
cleanse

The AYURVEDIC Path to Energy, Clarity, Wellness, and Your Best You

KIMBERLY LARSON

Foreword by Dr. Claudia Welch, MSOM

FAIR WINDS

{ PART I }

fundamentals of health & balance

PART II

cleansing for your body-mind type

FOREWORD

PUBLIC HEALTH IS THE SCIENCE AND ART of supporting the health and quality of life in a community. Though methods vary greatly among cultures, in general, public health practices aim to reach community members in a meaningful way—so that we as individuals change our behavior for the better. When we change, our communities change. When our communities change, our countries change. When our countries change, our world changes. Big change, as we so often hear, does indeed begin with each one of us. One of the most creative ways to reach individuals through public health is one I came across when I first studied health in India in 1988.

In India, if you are a very observant Hindu, you celebrate more religious holidays than there are days in a year. Every single day has particular significance according to its position in the lunar calendar. Celebrations of each day range from modest affairs with minimal rituals to elaborate celebrations in which millions of people participate. An individual's reason to celebrate might be to nourish one's relationship to spiritual practices, to maintain religious protocol, or simply to not irritate family or community sensibilities. But there are also positive large, "public health" scale, side effects of each individual's participation. Why? Dietary restrictions or observances often accompany holidays—typically in the form of a fast. For example, during a one-day holiday, a celebrant is enjoined to fast until the evening—and then break the fast only with certain simple foods. Giving the digestive system a mini break in this way provides a small, gentle cleanse. In addition to these shorter fasts and festivals, some festivals are held during seasonal transitions and require more lengthy fasts. During the nine-day holiday of Navaratri, for example, celebrants fast on either liquids or only certain easily-digestible foods. This holiday occurs multiple times a year, but the autumn and spring Navaratris are the most widely observed.

Because the benefits of occasional fasting, especially during seasonal transitions, has been well known to Ayurveda in India for millennia, it is widely believed that the dietary and lifestyle observances that accompany holidays—especially ones that occur during seasonal transitions—were consciously instituted to support public health. If people fast or simplify their diet during the changes of season—times when disease is more apt to be initiated—it allows the body and mind to gently cleanse and better adapt to the rhythms and realities of the new season. Tying these measures to religious holidays helped ensure that the population—whether educated about good health practices or not—would be obliged to adopt them and therefore potentially remain healthier. Although these practices may not be as strictly or widely practiced now, many Hindus still observe them. One recent example is that of India's Prime Minister Narendra Modi, who has, for decades, famously fasted on only liquids during Navaratri—even when it coincided with his maiden trip to the United States in the Fall of 2014, when he was sixty-four years old.

Though we in the West may not share the religion that initiated such fasts, we can still reap the benefits to mental, emotional, and spiritual health that these practices generate. Taking time to cleanse in a safe and gentle way, simplifying not only our diets but also fasting from the stimulation and demands of our daily responsibilities, allowing our attention to be stilled—or at least grow more still for a brief interlude—can refresh our energy, perspective, and relationship to life.

As individuals, we have the opportunity to educate ourselves about the wisdom of such practices and adopt them ourselves. This book can serve as a guide on how to calm and focus our attention, listen to and understand our bodies, simplify our diets, adopt gentle cleansing techniques, and internalize the value of doing so. Through these practices, our health can improve. Because our health also affects our families and our communities, we do change the world by changing ourselves.

So, happy holidays . . . whatever time of year you choose to celebrate good mental, spiritual, and physical health.

in love,

dr. claudia welch
doctor of oriental medicine

INTRODUCTION

hEALTH IS A STATE OF BEING that includes our physical, mental, and emotional selves. We can have good health in which the body feels strong and vibrant, the mind is calm, and the emotions are stable and positive, or we can have poor health in which all components of our being show signs of imbalance. Making a choice about your personal state of being can feel overwhelming, because the amount of information about health, diet, and lifestyle choices available to anyone with technology-savvy fingertips can be mind-boggling and conflicting.

Until I was introduced to the holistic system of medicine known as Ayurveda, I felt like I was randomly grasping at straws to choose which practices I should incorporate for my own health. But once I understood the intuitive, personalized Ayurvedic system, I could see that each diet, lifestyle, or cleanse out there is "healthy" for someone.

Cleansing is one practice that is often used to create better health—some people cleanse to lose weight, while others cleanse to improve the removal of byproducts from cellular metabolism, accumulations from poor diet, toxins in their food or environment, or qualities increased during each season of the year. However, this process intended to create better health can sometimes do the opposite.

I recall my first "cleanse," during which I drank only water for five days. A stranger told me how wonderful he felt after doing it, so I decided to try it. I did not have a framework to help me decide whether this would be a good idea for me; it definitely was not, and now, with knowledge of Ayurveda, I can see why. I was already thin and light in frame; it was a cooler than average autumn and I ended up chilled to the bone, ungrounded, and anxious from the lightening effects of the cleanse. This is an example of how practices meant to create better health can do the opposite if they are not chosen specifically for a person. The Ayurvedic framework can provide this personalized understanding.

After a decade as an Ayurvedic practitioner, I believe that people must address two factors before undertaking any cleanse. The first is to understand which diet will support health for you in your typical, everyday life and to use that knowledge to prepare food to nourish yourself. This baseline diet of personalized, healthful eating is important, because each one of us is different and therefore has different needs. We must meet those needs before we can prepare to undertake a cleanse. The second factor is to understand which type of cleanse is right for you, given your current state of health. The Ayurvedic principles explained in this book will provide the information needed to make knowledgeable decisions.

This book provides more than fifty recipes for personalized, healthful daily living as well as for times of cleansing. You can use the recipes for a seasonal everyday diet to maintain health by following the lightening recipes for spring, the cooling recipes for summer, and the grounding recipes for autumn. If you are feeling off or unhealthy, this book will help you determine your body type according to the Ayurvedic system and how your body may be out of balance. With that knowledge, you can create a daily diet to restore balance by choosing the modifications in each recipe that are appropriate for your body type. Part I of this book will give you the tools to understand your basic body-mind type and your current imbalance so that you can make good foundational choices about food.

You can also use these recipes when following the 31-day cleansing protocol, outlined in Part II. Designed to assist you in creating more awareness about food and re-learning how to eat every day, the protocol will improve your lifelong health and help you to make conscious choices as you prepare to cleanse. It will then guide you through a gentle Ayurvedic cleanse and describe how to end the cleanse easily and safely. During this process, the recipes you choose can help right any imbalance you might have, so that your food becomes like medicine.

All of this knowledge is useless if someone cannot apply it. Knowing what food is good for you is the first step, but finding simple, easy recipes and time to prepare them is another. These recipes are from my personal collection, created to inspire many clients over the years to care for themselves by cooking. My cooking tips eliminate 90 percent of the effort and time in the kitchen—and that is the "magic" that makes vibrant health attainable for even the busiest bee. I hope that this book and the tradition of Ayurveda inspire good health for you and your family for years to come.

fundamentals of health & balance

YOUR BODY IS SPEAKING TO you at every moment of every day. It is communicating each of its needs and challenges with simple, logical actions. Do you detect when your stomach tells you it is adequately full at each meal? Have you ever heard its tiny voice speaking to you, or do you just eat until discomfort arises and you feel heavy? Have you ever noticed the coating on your tongue when brushing your teeth? Did you know that the coating is your tongue revealing the state of your digestion, something that can help you decide which foods to eat each day? This is your body speaking in a language that most people have long forgotten, the innate wisdom that we all possess as infants but are not always encouraged to listen to as we grow into adults. The good news is that this language is easy to learn.

The colors and textures you see in your hair and skin when you peer into the mirror are hints of balance or imbalance. Your face—with its unique lines and creases, beauty marks and blemishes, and luster or lack thereof—tells a story of your health. Your eyes, often called the windows of the soul, share the truth of your being as emotions rise up and through them. Your tongue is a map of the internal world—the world of digestion, assimilation, and elimination. Your nails reveal secrets deep in your bones. Even your aches and pains are a cry: "Can you help? Here? There?" These are just some of the ways our bodies are always speaking to us.

Together, these bodily signs create a road map depicting the journey either away from balance or toward it. Before disease manifests, many road signs of warning may appear. Have you ever felt as if something in your body was just not right? Maybe you visited your doctor to report a series of seemingly unrelated symptoms, but the doctor found nothing wrong. These are the road signs. This is your intelligence speaking. Many ancient forms of medicine from India to China to Greece and beyond relied on reading and understanding these bodily signs to prevent and diagnose disease. If you are willing to look and listen carefully, you can understand your body's language and make prevention your key to health.

Ayurveda is a common-sense medicine we need in modern society. Originating more than 5,000 years ago in India, Ayurveda is a traditional medical science based on natural principles that apply to all life. It not only recognizes the uniqueness of each individual but also outlines principles that support better health for each body-mind type— the physiological and psychological characteristics of an individual that

Ayurveda categorizes into three main types, which are described in detail in chapter 2. With the individual as its focus, Ayurveda offers a model of prevention-based medicine that many cultures lack today—a true system of health care, not just sick care! Although Ayurveda prioritizes self-observation and self-care practices to foster good health, Ayurveda also has many specialized branches such as internal medicine, surgery, pediatrics, psychology, and rejuvenation to improve health when we are sick or injured.

According to Ayurveda, health care has four simple steps.

1. Learn the basic principles that apply to all life, so that you can see yourself and the world around you clearly.
2. Use these principles to determine your body-mind type, and then follow diet and lifestyle practices appropriate for your type.
3. Learn to attune to the cycles of nature, living in harmony with the seasons and thus maximizing your energy.
4. Cleanse the body regularly and follow up with a period of rejuvenation to remove any unhealthy accumulation before it can develop into a problem.

Part I of this book walks you through these four steps; Part II lays out a simple 31-day protocol to prepare your body to go in to and ease out of a gentle Ayurvedic cleanse.

the essence of ayurveda

INTELLIGENCE IS YOUR BIRTHRIGHT. Your body is a miracle, and every one of the trillions of cells working together in your body is intelligent. They all know exactly how to function, which nutrients to use, and how to cooperate with one another. Ayurveda, which translates as the "science of life," is based on a firm understanding of this intelligence, and the classic textbooks of Ayurveda state that disease often begins when we ignore the body's wisdom.

Your body is logical in every action and reaction, and it speaks out against any action that does not foster good health. Sometimes it speaks quietly, such as through a coating on your tongue, and other times it speaks loudly, for example, through the symptoms of a hangover. If you ignore this intelligence too long, it will eventually respond with "dis-ease." Disease is not a mysterious or instantaneous event; rather, it comes from a progression of imbalances that accumulate in a logical and natural order over time.

It is easier to care for one's health than to cure a disease. One of Ayurveda's goals, therefore, is to prevent disease by encouraging individuals to take personal responsibility for their health. A daily practice of caring for oneself as a good mother cares for her child—with healthy food, proper exercise, protection against the elements of nature, restful sleep, nurturing touch, and abundant love—is a big step toward ensuring a healthy body and mind. We each have a responsibility to be a good parent

PRAJNAPARADHA: "CRIMES AGAINST WISDOM"

Disease may flourish when we when we ignore the intelligence of our body. We ignore the intelligence of our body when we: (a) don't know how listen to it in the first place; or (b) know how to listen to it, but ignore what it is saying.

Our bodies are composed of a mind-bogglingly complicated bunch of systems, genes, hormones, microbiomes, emotions, thoughts, and organs. To know what is going on in our body at any given time requires that we pay close attention to the signals it is constantly producing—signals like anxiety, thirst, fatigue, hunger, lack of appetite, constipation, loose stools, gas, bloating, heartburn, and sensations of heaviness, dullness, excessive lightness, and dizziness—or even the feeling that everything is perfect. When we practice paying attention to these signals and how their presence reflects our environment, diet, relationships, emotions, and lifestyle, we become more adept at recognizing, interpreting and responding to the signals in a manner that fosters good health. —DR. CLAUDIA WELCH

to ourselves so that we can contribute our best potential to our families, our communities, and the world.

LONGEVITY

According to Ayurveda, the body is the vehicle for our energy, our minds, and even our souls. It is difficult to focus on anything else when the body is sick or experiencing pain. Like a wounded animal that instinctively hides to protect itself, we seek shelter when we are sick by turning inward to focus our energy on healing. If the body is not sound, there is little energy available for learning, creativity, growth, or transformation. Imbalance and illness limit our ability to expand our lives beyond our own immediate physical needs, and this limitation prohibits expansion of our minds, hearts, and spirits.

Longevity is one of Ayurveda's primary aims, so people

have a lifetime of opportunity to develop a spiritual practice that takes them beyond the physical existence of the body. Ayurveda's goal is one hundred healthy years for each person. For many this goal may sound unrealistic, because many people now reach their eighties, nineties, or are even older, but most are not healthy. This does not need to be the case.

The process of aging is universal; we will all pass on from this life one day and most of us will grow old first. But the symptoms of "aging" have more to do with the relative state of balance in the body than with physical age. Dan Buettner, in collaboration with *National Geographic* and the National Institute on Aging, studied areas of the world where centenarians are common. In the book *Blue Zones: 9 Lessons For Living Longer from the People Who've Lived the Longest,* he reported the common threads in communities where people live to age one hundred at a rate ten times greater than the global average, where life expectancy is typically twelve years longer than the worldwide average, and where the rate of middle-age mortality is a fraction of that in other places. He found diet and lifestyle factors to be the most substantial differences.

Genetics does play a role in the rate at which one's body shows signs of aging—some people have gray hair at age twenty, while others have a full head of dark hair at eighty—but it is not the only factor. The degenerative symptoms and diseases typically associated with old age can occur at a young age if the body is severely imbalanced. For example, arthritis of the hands is commonly seen in the elderly, but it could also manifest in a young person who uses his or her hands in a repetitive and excessive way, as a welder does. According to Ayurveda, the reverse is also true: The body can remain soft, supple, and flexible into old age when people perform proper self-care and maintenance throughout their lives.

DEFINITION OF HEALTH

Health is a lot like a garden. The seeds of genetics and our natural intelligence carry our potential. When planted in fertile soil with enough water and nutrients, good health sprouts. It requires the hard work of daily care and the diligence of maintenance to help it continue to grow into its fullness. Nature provides the setting and ingredients, but we must put forth the effort if we want to harvest the bounty of good health.

One obstacle to this bounty is that many cultures define "health" solely as the absence of disease. We all know long-term cigarette smokers, survivors of heart attacks, and individuals with diabetes who feel "healthy" despite obvious manifestations of disease. Conversely, many individuals feel "unhealthy" with unexplained symptoms of imbalance, but their doctors report them to be "normal." So what is health?

Ayurveda defines health in an extremely different way:

> A person who has balanced physiological forces, balanced metabolic fire, properly formed tissues and waste products, who is established in Self, and whose being (mind-body-soul-senses) is full of bliss, is a healthy individual.
>
> —translation from *Charaka Samhita*, an ancient Ayurvedic textbook

AYURVEDIC TOOLBOX: GET OUT

Observe: Cultivate the skill of observing qualities in yourselves and the environment.

Understand: Use the principles of Ayurveda to understand what these qualities mean for your body-mind type and current imbalance.

Transform: Make intelligent choices based on this knowledge to transform your health.

twenty qualities

— or ten pairs of opposites —

PAIRS	IN NATURE	IN THE BODY
Light/Heavy	dandelion seed/boulder	underweight/ overweight
Sharp/Dull	thorn/mud	sharp pain/ dull sensation
Cold/Hot	winter/ summer	cold extremities such as hands or feet/fever
Dry/Oily	desert/ rain forest	dry/oily skin
Rough/Smooth	bark/leaf	rough/smooth nails or hair
Dense/Liquiad; Amorphous	earth/water	muscles/blood
Hard/Soft	rocks/moss	bones/fat
Mobile/Static; Stable	wind/earth	racing thoughts/ stable focus
Subtle (having little to no physical mass)/ Gross (having solid bulk or physical mass)	air/wood	emotions/flesh
Sticky/Clear	tree sap/air	mucus/ tears

This definition provides clear indicators of health. It offers criteria for measuring it and uplifts the truth that our natural state of health can bring bliss on all levels. Ayurveda is clear that health can be established only if it includes all aspects of ourselves—body, mind, soul, and senses. This is a rare jewel, but it is attainable.

Ayurveda provides a unique framework that is proactive, engaged, and tailored to the individual. It provides tools for self-assessment, systematic steps for cultivating health, and individual guidelines for maintaining it, based on three body-mind types. The steps to cultivate health can be summed up with three actions: observe, understand, transform. See the sidebar on page 17 for details.

QUALITIES

Every plant, every animal, and every substance on our planet has unique qualities. Water, for example, is cold unless heated by the sun or a fire. Water is heavy, and thus flows downward with gravity. Fire, on the other hand, is hot and light, and its flames flare upward. Each of these qualities exists as one of a pair of opposites: hot or cold, light or heavy, smooth or rough, moist or dry.

We are constantly using these pairs to maintain balance, or homeostasis, in our bodies. In the heat of summer we seek out a cool drink, a shady spot to sit, or a fan, because opposites balance each other. This is one of the first lessons we learn as infants. Even a young child learns to seek out the warmth of a mother's arms or a blanket when cold. This innate knowledge grows over time as we begin to understand the world around us, but the first step is learning to observe these qualities.

OBSERVATION WALK

Take a walk in nature and try to observe qualities in each unique element you notice. Bring the list of pairs on page 18 and make sure to find at least one example in nature of each quality. Start by describing the weather, the geography, and the season. Look at the trees: Describe their structure, bark, and leaves with these pairs of opposites. Notice that different species of trees have slightly different qualities. Observe the earth and any plants, bodies of water, and animals you encounter. Notice any qualities that are present in abundance in the area.

FINDING BALANCE

The principle of opposites is constantly at play in nature: The cool of night follows the heat of day; a dry season follows the rainy season; and the cool of fall follows the heat of summer. These vacillations between opposite qualities create a natural rhythm that brings balance to the environment. All of the qualities manifest at a proper place and time.

Our bodies also have a natural rhythm. Each quality must exist in the proper amount for balance to exist. For example, the hot, sharp, and penetrating qualities of the digestive acids in your stomach require sufficient cool, oily, and sticky mucus to protect the lining of the stomach. If the proper balance is not maintained, an ulcer could result. All imbalances in the body follow a logical progression. In the case of an ulcer, you might first feel heat in the stomach, then a burning sensation or acid reflux, and if it continues for a long time, pain as the heating acids ultimately eat through the lining of the stomach. When the natural balance is disrupted, we must act.

If you are feeling hot, you can encourage a return to balance when you apply cold in any form, such as exposure to a cold climate, cold foods or drinks; a cool shower or bath; an herb with cooling properties; or a cooling breath or yoga pose. We may have numerous options, because everything in the universe has qualities, so anything that has the cooling quality could be a potential medicine to restore balance. In the previous example of an ulcer, a cooling diet would help to soothe the burning heat in the stomach and restore balance, especially if someone adopts this diet at the first signs of heat.

Ayurveda uses this principle of opposites at every level of the body to maintain health. Every food and drink you consume has an effect on the body. Every thought and emotion you experience affects your body. Seasons and climates do as well. Exercise or lack of exercise, self-care or lack of self-care, and sleep or lack of sleep all have an impact. The universe is full of potential for healing. All we need to do is observe our predominant qualities, understand how they are affecting us, and transform ourselves by applying the principle of opposites. Ayurveda recognizes that each body is different, so the recipe for health it prescribes requires an individual analysis, which is explained in the next chapter.

understanding your body-mind type

aYURVEDA USES THIS INDIVIDUALITY as a basis for understanding health. Each of us requires different foods, exercises, activities, and daily practices to maintain health or restore it when we lose balance. Understanding your body-mind type can empower you to make choices every day to help improve your health even if you have a chronic condition.

Ancient seers, or *rishis*, observed nature and noticed that the human being is a microcosm of the macrocosm. The forces present in nature are parallel to forces that shape our internal universe. Three fundamental principles govern movement, structure, and transformation. The principle of movement is like a wind or breeze, the principle of structure is like earth, and the principle of transformation is like fire. These three principles are cogs in the machine of creation and in the body and mind. When they are associated with the internal organization of the body and mind we call them *doshas*. In Sanskrit, they are *Vata*, *Kapha*, and *Pitta*, respectively. For the purposes of this book, we will associate these principles with the body-mind types Breeze, Mountain, and Fire, respectively.

The dosha that is predominant in you creates your body-mind type. Predominance in Vata, or Breeze, creates a body-mind type that is mobile, variable, light like the wind, and as delicate as a flower. Predominance of Kapha, or Mountain, creates a body-mind type that is sturdy and strong like a mountain. Predominance of Pitta,

THE FIVE ELEMENTS

These elements observed by the ancient seers are the basic building blocks of life and compose all matter in the universe. A combination of two of the five elements makes up each dosha.

Ether (space) + Air = Vata dosha • Fire + Water = Pitta dosha • Water + Earth = Kapha dosha

See page 200 of the appendix for a more detailed description of the five elements.

or Fire, creates an individual who is active, driven, and full of fire and heat. Each of these three types possesses specific qualities and actions that distinguish them from one another, and they require different self-care routines.

VATA DOSHA

— *or the breeze type* —

In Ayurveda, the internal principle of movement is called *vata dosha*, from the Sanskrit root *va* meaning "to move." It is a combination of all the qualities of space (ether) and air elements. Air moving through a space creates a wind. The central nervous system controls all internal movements, from the conscious contracting of muscles to the unconscious beating of the heart. Thus, vata dosha is intimately linked with the nervous system.

When predominant, vata will manifest a physical body that is light and thin with little fat stores. Because of this, and because fat in the form of a myelin sheath is the insulator of every nerve fiber, the nervous system is not well insulated in vata-predominant individuals. This makes the vata individual particularly sensitive, like an exposed electrical wire. The Ayurvedic saying, "Treat a vata like a delicate flower" reflects this sensitivity.

qualities

Cold, dry, light, rough, mobile, subtle, and sensitive are all qualities of the Breeze type, but the most pronounced is mobile. The dominant quality of Breeze is movement. Consider the incredibly vital role movement plays in our organisms: The constant and consistent movement of our hearts, breath, peristalsis, urine, sweat, lymphatic fluid, cellular respiration, blood, oxygen, nutrition into cells, waste out of cells, cerebrospinal fluid, thoughts, and attention all play nuanced, powerful roles in health. When this movement is natural, relaxed, regular, and flowing, we experience health. When it is too fast, too slow, or otherwise thwarted, we experience disturbance.

Our internal rhythms and movements track and respond to the external environment. To better understand this, picture a flower in bloom in a meadow. As the sun rises, her petals open in response. She turns toward the sun and follows it along its path across the sky. A gentle wind blows and she waves. Stronger winds blow and she bends. A bee lands on her, then later a butterfly. She is not only subjected to and affected by external movement but also to her own mobile responses to the environment. Her natural internal movement influences how she follows the path of the sun and opens and closes her petals; her internal responses to the interactions with the bee and the

breeze type

ACTION: movement

ELEMENTS: air and space,
like the wind or breeze

QUALITIES: cold, dry, light, rough,
mobile, subtle, and clear

BODY FRAME: thin, narrow, and light

MOVEMENTS: fast, erratic,
or variable

butterfly; and the flow of nutrients, sunlight, and waste throughout her organism.

Like the flower, we human beings are constantly in motion—a combination of our internal physiological motion and our responses to the environment. When the mobile quality is balanced, we can stay focused, have routine times for bowel habits, our heartbeats are regular, and other processes that motion governs are healthy. Although the mobile quality is a defining feature of Vata, the other qualities associated with this type tend to affect and afflict Breeze types also. They tend to be quite thin, due to the light quality; have dry or rough skin, bowels, and hair, due to the dry and rough quality; and have active imaginations and inner lives, due to the subtle quality that creates an expansive mind.

physical constitution

An individual with a Breeze body type may be very tall or very short, thin, lanky, and sometimes has asymmetric features. The person's frame tends to be narrow, thin, and light, with a small bone structure, light muscle mass, and little body fat. The light and dry qualities of the Breeze keep these individuals thin despite how much food they eat, and it is often difficult for them to gain weight. Without much insulation, they can easily feel sensitive to cold, wind, dry weather, and even to too much stimulation from the environment or surroundings. Facial features are small, thin, or delicate, with quick or frequent movements such as blinking often. Their skin, hair, and nails may show signs of rough and dry qualities, and the qualities of mobility and variability are pronounced in most of their actions and preferences.

nature

Because movement is the most distinguishing factor for this type, Breeze individuals move fast, walk fast, and talk fast. Like a little butterfly or a hummingbird, they move quickly from one thing to the next—ideas, thoughts, projects, conversations, and even relationships. They often enjoy a variety of physical and social activities, travel, and new experiences. Ideas and thoughts flow through their minds easily, like a constant wind giving them great creative powers. This expansive ability of the mind influences many Breeze types to become musicians, artists, or writers. It is often difficult for these individuals to slow down their bodies and minds, as this quality of mobility permeates their lives and their love of variability may keep them from establishing solid, lasting routines.

KAPHA DOSHA

— or the mountain type —

Kapha is the Ayurvedic term used to describe the physiological principles of structure and lubrication considered the body's glue, or cohesive force. The solid structures of the body such as bones, joints, muscles, and fat, as well as the liquid or lubricating substances such as saliva, mucus, plasma, lymph, and synovial fluid in the joints are composed of the building blocks of kapha. The word *kapha* translates as "that which flourishes by water" or "that which holds things together."

qualities

The qualities of the earth element—hard, dense, solid, and stable—combined with the qualities of water element—liquid, soft, fluid, and cold—describe all of the body's physical structures, from bones and muscles to lymph and plasma. An individual who has a predominance of the kapha dosha will have abundant body mass and lubrication, which form a strong, solid structure not easily disturbed by external forces, much like a mountain.

Think of the qualities of a majestic mountain: large, solid, stable, heavy, dense, and hard. The mountain seems immovable. Does the wind change the mountain at all? Yes, but not the way it affects a flower. We know that mountains move and change over time, but gradually. The forces of nature erode a mountain, but it takes thousands of years. Now picture the mountain more closely; imagine a stream trickling from the cloud-covered top and meandering down through cold, mossy rocks. Consider the qualities you see here: moist, smooth, soft, cold, and slow. All of the qualities listed for both the sturdy earth and softer water elements compose the Mountain body type.

physical constitution

The physical constitution of a Mountain is large, solid, and stable, with good strength, stamina, and resilience. The Mountain's bone structure, muscle mass, and store of body fat are larger than that of the other body types, and the incredible insulation this creates makes the Mountain seem barely affected by heat or cold, hunger or thirst, and even lack of sleep or excessive activity. People with this body type move slowly in all aspects of their lives and enjoy the comfort of routines that are reliably stable and long lasting. The heaviness and inertia they can accumulate tend to make change and variability challenging. A slower metabolism makes it easy for them to store up excesses but difficult to lose weight or clear out accumulations, such as mucus. Their facial features are large and broad, with smooth, moist skin, abundant long eyelashes, full lips, and a thick, luxurious head of hair. They are sturdy and stable in their physical bodies and in their routines, thoughts, and emotions.

mountain type

ACTIONS: **structure and lubrication**

ELEMENTS: **earth and water**

QUALITIES: **cool, moist, heavy, stable, smooth, oily, dense, liquid, hard, soft, gross, dull, and sticky**

BODY FRAME: **large, heavy, and dense**

MOVEMENTS: **slow and steady**

nature

The nature of the Mountain type is to hold. They physically hold on to more muscle mass, weight, and moisture than other types do, but they also excel at holding on to money, relationships, and love. Their reliable, steady emotions make them wonderful friends, confidants, and teachers, able to offer sympathy and empathy with ease and bring comfort to others. Comfort plays a key role in their lives, especially at home—where they often like to stay, enjoying the leisure of reading, cooking, or relaxing. A lavishly comfortable bed, sitting area, or car may be a sign of the Mountain type. Strong memory is another asset of the Mountain even though this type may take longer than others to learn or gather information. Like elephants, Mountains "never forget," which serves them well in the academic and business worlds but can be challenging in their personal and emotional lives, because they may hold on to old emotions, experiences, and grudges. When they are balanced, they can easily forgive and lavish love.

The Mountain and the Breeze look like opposites in most ways: One is rarely affected by the external environment, the other constantly overwhelmed by it; one is immovable or slow, the other is in constant motion and fast. The two types share one major quality: cold. Neither the Breeze nor the Mountain generates heat; their nature is cool.

PITTA DOSHA
— or the fire type —

The center of our solar system is the intensely hot star we call the sun; the center of a cell is a metabolic command center called the nucleus; and the center of the human body holds the acids and digestive enzymes we call our digestive fire, or *agni*. Fire in all its forms is the universal principle that creates transformation. The ancient Ayurvedic rishis clearly perceived this transformational internal force and named it *pitta* from the root verb *tapa* meaning "to heat."

qualities

Pitta dosha combines qualities of the fire element with qualities of the water element, resulting in a combination of qualities: oily, sharp, hot, light, spreading, and liquid. Pitta is present in the stomach region for transformation of food and in the brain to transform stimuli from the sense organs into thoughts, feelings, and emotions. Each cell must have adequate pitta to carry out cellular metabolism and direct proper functioning of its parts. A pitta-predominant individual will exhibit this fire in all areas of the physical body and the mind.

The Fire type, unlike the Breeze and Mountain types, is inherently hot. Picture yourself sitting next to a roaring campfire as it lights up and warms the surrounding area. Observe the continuous movement. Notice how easily the flames build and spread, transforming the wood and everything it touches. Know that if you touch its flame you, too, will feel the fire's sharp bite.

physical constitution

The Fire type is medium in size and build: medium height, muscle mass, and amount of body fat. The face has sharp, medium-size features. The manifestations of Fire characteristics are visible everywhere on the body. The skin is sensitive to the sun, fair, freckled, and slightly oily. The cheeks are rosy, the lips are red, and a brightness or lightness illuminates the eyes. The internal heat of transformation keeps the Fire type's body and mind hot, even in a cold season or climate. The digestive fire is strong, allowing Fire individuals to eat heartily without gaining unneeded weight.

nature

The mind of a Fire individual mirrors a strong appetite. People with this body type have a passion for knowledge, experience, and intensity. Fire is a transformative force, and in their mind it creates a sharp intellect with a desire for understanding. The questions of why and how are of utmost importance. Their sharp minds naturally create order and organization, allowing them to see patterns and big pictures, be detail-oriented (sometimes to the point of perfectionism), and good at strategizing and coordinating when they are in balance. The Fire type is the epitome of Type A personality in our multitasking culture. This fire can fuel mental activities and work, intense physical activities (like skydiving, rock climbing, or running a marathon), and passionate emotions. The fiery emotions of frustration, anger, and rage can flare up when the Fire is out of

balance. Burnout can also be a real consequence of an imbalance of too much intensity or activity.

Now the important question remains: Which type are you? A Breeze, a Fire, or a Mountain? You will most likely see in yourself aspects of all three types, because we must have all three natural forces to exist. Still, most of us have a strong tendency toward one or two of these categories. According to Ayurveda, each person, from the moment of birth, is a unique combination of these three forces. The resulting combination is known as one's "constitution." Although most people have a strong predominance in one or two of the three doshas, an individual may have all three in equal amount. Each type has its strengths and weaknesses, and the foundation of health lies in knowing your personal combination.

The word *dosha* actually translates as "that which goes

DELICATE YET STRONG

People with a predominance of Fire encounter unique circumstances that the other two types do not. Although their intellectual abilities and ambitions are especially strong, their physical constitution can be somewhat delicate. For example, though competitive and slow to admit or even recognize it, they will indeed tire from strong physical labor more quickly than the Mountain type—especially if they are laboring in hot weather. The Fire type tends to identify with the strength of their own intellect and ambitions and may believe they are also physically strong. Because they respect their ambitions and intellect more than their body, they often pursue their ambitions despite their body telling them for years that it can't keep up. It is not uncommon for the Fire type to disbelieve or ignore the delicacy of their physical constitution until it screams at them, forcing them to slow down. It is therefore a good practice for Fire types to surrender to the pace of their bodies—a practice that does not come easily—if they want to maintain physical health as well as intellectual prowess. This first requires that they are in touch with the real pace of their body, which requires a practice of internal reflection. —DR. CLAUDIA WELCH

fire type

ACTION: transformation

ELEMENTS: fire and water

QUALITIES: hot, light, sharp, mobile, liquid, and spreading

BODY FRAME: medium

MOVEMENTS: moderate pace and deliberate

Sometimes it is helpful to answer the Constitution Checklist from the perspective of your childhood, given that your constitution is the unique combination of these doshas at the moment of your birth. Occasionally, our true nature is masked by the imbalances we have accumulated over the years.

Take your time when filling out the Constitution Checklist. Consider your characteristics as a whole throughout your lifetime. If you find that your answers are dramatically different from the answers you would give based on your childhood self, create two columns and answer one for each, to see how they compare.

THE BREEZE
— in and out of balance —

out of balance," which describes the aspect we often see most clearly. For this reason, Ayurveda seeks to first determine your constitution, called *prakriti*, and then your current state of imbalance, called *vikriti*.

Filling out the Constitution Checklist on page 196 is one way to determine which doshas are predominant for you. Clear observation is the first step. This requires an honest assessment of your qualities, a process that can be difficult at first. It may be helpful to fill out the checklist with a friend or family member who can give you perspective. The checklist covers physical attributes of your body, mental tendencies, likes and dislikes, and even emotional patterns. If you find that you have a combination of qualities from more than one type for one category, mark each one. For example, if your skin is both dry and fair, then place a check next to each statement. The goal is to find an overall trend, though many people have a sense of their type before they go through the list. When you finish, total the number of checks in each category to see where your predominance resides.

The strengths of any body-mind type are present when an individual is in balance, and the weaknesses show up when she is out of balance. The Breeze individual exhibits creativity, clarity, imagination, and love of diversity when in balance. Healthy functions encompass all conscious and unconscious movements in the body, as well as all muscular movements, as described here:

- ❖ Inward movement or intake: sensory stimuli, mental processes, inhalation, and swallowing;
- ❖ Upward movement: exhalation, coughing, speaking/expression, hiccuping, and vomiting;
- ❖ Digestive movement: coordinating the process of digestion and movement through the digestive tract;
- ❖ Circulatory movement: heart pulsation, movement of blood, and lymphatic movement; and
- ❖ Downward movement: elimination of wastes and reproductive fluids, expelling the fetus, and grounding.

Kapha

THE MOUNTAIN
— in and out of balance —

These movements are all necessary to keep the body at optimum health, and, when in balance, the Breeze individual experiences each type of movement in proper proportions.

When Breeze individuals are out of balance, the natural predominant qualities—cold, light, dry, rough, mobile, subtle, and clear—will accumulate. This means someone may feel internally cold, have cold extremities, and could develop an aversion to wind or cold. Signs of imbalance manifest as dark discolorations of the body or wastes, such as in the eyes, nails, skin, urine, or feces. Skin, hair, nails, lips, mouth, nose, eyes, ears, joints, or the colon may become dry, because these are parts of the body that require fluids and mucus to function properly.

For example, synovial fluid in the joints is the natural lubrication that eases movement, and when the dry quality affects these fluids, one can hear cracking and popping sounds with joint movement. If that persists for some time, pain and discomfort may follow, eventually limiting the range of motion in the joint and possibly creating deformities in its shape and structure. If the dry quality affects the colon, the mucus lining will lose its natural lubrication and the stools will become hard, leading to constipation.

Excessive mobility can lead to muscular twitches, spasms, irregular bowel movements, or a busy or scattered mind that cannot stop, even to sleep (insomnia). Accumulation of vata in the colon, considered its homesite in the body, can contribute to constipation, pain in the low back, hips, or thighs, eventually leading to sciatica. The variability or weakness of digestive strength produces gas, bloating, and other kinds of abdominal discomfort. Too much lightness can manifest as insomnia, a light-headed or ungrounded feeling, anxiety, or nervousness. Emotionally, an imbalance can also create fear, instability, or insecurity. Throughout the book, we categorize all of these as Breeze imbalances.

Strong, sturdy Mountain individuals are grounded, loving, compassionate, and reliable when in balance, making them good teachers and caregivers. Healthy functions include providing raw materials that build all the tissues of the body and lubricate or insulate these parts of the body:

- ⁜ Stomach: to aid digestion;
- ⁜ Lungs and heart: to reduce friction from the constant movement of these organs and counteract the dryness of the air we breathe;
- ⁜ Joints: to allow fluid movements;
- ⁜ Mouth: to allow taste by the tongue, the act of swallowing, and the start of the process of digestion; and
- ⁜ Brain and nervous system: to produce the cerebrospinal fluid, the myelin sheath, and white matter of the brain

We need adequate substance to build and maintain all body tissue, to lubricate the body and ensure ease of movement, and to protect the tissues and organs from damage. When in balance, the Mountain easily supplies the proper amount of materials for each function and gives strength to the body.

When out of balance, the Mountain individual's natural qualities—cool, heavy, smooth, oily, dense, liquid, soft, dull, stable, gross, and sticky—will create excess accumulations in the body and mind. In the body, heaviness, weight gain, lethargy, fluid retention, edema, or nausea may manifest. A Mountain imbalance might be more noticeable during a woman's menses, when all of those symptoms may affect her at the same time. A dull or cool digestive fire can create slow digestion or allow excess mucus to accumulate in the lungs, sinuses, stools, or stomach, which is considered the homesite of kapha in the body. Thick, white accumulations or discharges show imbalance, and accumulations of soft or hard masses such as fatty tumors, cysts, and cancerous or benign growths are common. Emotionally, the excess stable quality may turn into attachment, stubbornness, or greed when imbalanced.

As an example of how imbalance progresses, dull digestive fire could lead to overproduction of mucus in the stomach, creating nausea and a feeling of heaviness. These symptoms might lead a Mountain individual to rest in the daytime instead of being physically active—activity is important to counteract their stability and density. The accumulation might extend to the lungs, where it reduces the intake of oxygen and energy, creating lethargy and more inactivity, which may eventually result in weight gain, fluid retention, swollen joints, and the inability of the body to efficiently rid itself of wastes. This may also affect a person's emotional health, creating a sense of depression. Throughout the book, we categorize these as Mountain imbalances.

THE HOUSE OF THE BODY

Imagine building a house:

Kapha (Mountain) functions as the principle of **structure and stability** and supplies the raw materials to build the foundation, structure, walls, floors, insulation, and every fixture and feature of the house. In the body, the gross physical components are bones, muscles, fat, organs, and fluids. Building a house or a body requires gross, physical "stuff," and the qualities of the Mountain type reflect this.

Pitta (Fire) is the heating system of the house and the body. The fire in the kitchen's stove transforms raw materials of food into easily digested meals, just as the fire in the belly is responsible for internal transformation of various foods into a substance that can nourish every cell of the body. Pitta is the principle providing for both **temperature regulation and transformation**. In the house, the heating system consists of a source and pipes—not as much physical stuff, but extremely important to the house. The qualities of the Fire type are subtler in nature than the Mountain's qualities.

Vata (Breeze) is the electrical system, which resembles the sensory impulses and the nervous system in our bodies where all **movement** originates. Its qualities are the most subtle and mobile in the house.

From the gross to the subtle, all parts of the house are equally important, just as the three doshas are needed in the body in the proper proportion.

THE FIRE
— in or out of balance —

The positive qualities associated with a Fire individual who is in balance are organization, order, clear communication, and a sharp intellect. Healthy functions are related to temperature regulation and transformation: transformation of food into energy, data into information, information into wisdom, and raw elements into biologically refined substances that nourish the body. These functions are particularly active in these parts of the body:

‍   ÷ Stomach and small intestines (considered the homesite of pitta in the body), as digestive enzymes;
   ÷ Liver, as bile;
   ÷ Skin, for temperature regulation;
   ÷ Eyes, for visual perception; and
   ÷ Heart-mind, for digestion of sensory input into thoughts, feelings, and emotions.

When the Fire is in balance, proper amounts of heat, acids, and enzymes are present to carry out natural functions.

When out of balance, the heating qualities of the Fire start to consume the body and mind. Hot or burning sensations, redness, inflammation, yellow discolorations, and sharp sensations of pain can manifest anywhere in the body, including the eyes, stomach, and joints. The stools may become soft or liquid and dark yellow in color. The yellow discoloration of eyes, nails, teeth, skin, or any other body part or waste product reflects an imbalance. The skin may become sensitive and prone to inflammation, resulting in acne, hives, or rashes. Digestive issues include loose stools, acid reflux, heartburn, gastritis, gastric ulcers, pain, or burning sensations. Fire individuals may experience excessive thirst, and the heated emotions of anger, frustration, rage, and jealousy may flare up. Throughout the book, we categorize these as Fire imbalances.

After you have filled out the Constitution Checklist (see page 196), fill out the Imbalance Checklist (see page 197). Answer according to how you are feeling **in this moment**—not your past history or your overall trends. This will give you more-accurate information on your current state of imbalance. The imbalance that you are experiencing may or may not be similar to your constitution. An individual with a Breeze constitution may easily be swayed into a Breeze imbalance, because they already have an abundance of those qualities, but that is not always the case. A person with a Breeze constitution can have a Mountain imbalance from having a sedentary lifestyle over a period of years. A person with a Fire constitution could "blow out" their fire from too much activity or movement, resulting in a Breeze imbalance—or that same excessive movement could "ignite an inferno," resulting in a Fire imbalance. It is important to accurately discern both constitution and imbalance separately.

"Let food be thy medicine, and medicine be thy food."

—Hippocrates, Father of Modern Medicine

CHAPTER THREE

foods for balance

PERSONAL TRANSFORMATION BEGINS with knowledge. You have observed yourself and your natural qualities, filled out the Constitution Checklist and Imbalance Checklist (see pages 196 and 197) to determine and understand your unique body-mind type and imbalance, and now you are ready to make choices that can transform your health. Food can, and should be medicine—this has been the basis of most health-care systems throughout time. Dr. Mark Hyman, in a TED talk on functional medicine, states that poor lifestyle choices, including diet, cause the majority of chronic, degenerative diseases, making them preventable. That means millions of individuals could have avoided suffering if they had the knowledge to transform themselves with their choices and acted on it. Luckily, you can gain this knowledge and transform yourself and your health. Are you ready to start?

FOOD-MEDICINE

Understanding what qualities are in the foods you eat is essential for health. Food builds every cell of your body. What you eat is without a doubt one of the most important decisions you make every day, though no single diet is right for every person. Ayurveda has pointed out two simple principles you can use to determine which foods are appropriate for you: the "principle of opposites" and "like increases like." These principles are two sides of the same coin: Similar qualities increase and opposite qualities decrease.

In general, we want to eat foods that have qualities opposite of those qualities that are high in our bodies. For example, if I feel too heavy, I want foods that are light in quality. If I feel too hot, I want cooling foods. Whatever type you are, you will tend to have an excess of that type's qualities. For example, the Breeze individual is cold, dry, and light in nature and therefore finds comfort and balance eating warm, moist, and heavy foods. The Mountain is cold, heavy, and moist in nature and needs foods that are hot, light, and dry to help bring balance. Finally, the Fire individual exhibits hot and light qualities and finds balance when eating foods that are cool and heavy. And though your constitution has a bit of each type, by following a diet designed for your predominant type, you can improve your balance and health. Like increases like, so if you are already cold and you eat ice cream, the logical effect is that you get colder. We can use this principle—and the principle of opposites—to make good decisions about our diet every day.

Whenever you eat something, the qualities in that food permeate your body. When you eat a chili pepper, the sharp, hot qualities first hit the tongue, then a burning sensation happens in your throat and stomach, and finally sweat begins to pour off of your brow. The heat of the pepper transfers to your being; you become hot like the pepper. To the Breeze individual, who is sensitive and delicate like a flower, this chili pepper might feel painful and overwhelming to the senses. To the sturdy, well-insulated Mountain, however, it might feel like a mild warming action that is a welcome change from his natural cool state. To a Fire type, the stimulation and rush of endorphins that follow might be exhilarating, but the stomach and digestive tract may continue to burn for days afterward. Food

POTENCY OF FOODS

Ayurveda classifies each food by its heating or cooling influence on the body. With some sensitivity or practice of awareness, you can feel this potency, or *virya*, in the stomach. The term *virya* can also be translated as "strength," "energy," or "power." The potency of some foods can be easily discerned, such as with a cucumber, which feels cool and juicy in the mouth as well as the stomach. But some foods might be harder to "feel"—some grains, for example, are heating and some are cooling. A foods list can initially help give you some perspective, but ideally you will learn to listen to your body and feel for yourself. Check out Dr. Vasant Lad's *Ayurveda: The Science of Self-Healing* for a detailed foods list.

chosen with awareness can be medicine, but food chosen without awareness can be poison.

the six tastes

You can see the importance of observing two sets of qualities: those that are increased in you and those inherent in your food choices. Once again, the Ayurvedic tool to get you *out* of old habits and into new, healthier ones relies on observation. We also have another sense that helps us with the important job of choosing foods to be our medicine: taste.

Nature has designed a simple system of tastes to help us understand which foods will benefit us. According to Ayurveda, food has six tastes: sweet, sour, salty, pungent, bitter, and astringent. Each taste has one or more specific actions on the body, in addition to the heating or cooling effect initially felt on the tongue and in the stomach.

Sweet taste is present in fruits and some vegetables such as carrots and beets; in concentrated form in honey and sugar; and more subtly in grains, particularly rice. **Sour** shows up in citrus fruits or unripe berries and in fermented items like vinegar, yogurt, hard cheeses, and cultured or pickled vegetables. **Salty** taste is naturally inherent in seaweed and all varieties of salt. **Pungent**, also called "spicy," is the heating sensation from garlic, onions, peppers, and spices such as black pepper, chili pepper, and paprika. **Bitter** is the flavor of dark leafy greens. It is present to some degree in all green vegetables, but is also the roasted flavor we love in dark chocolate and coffee. Finally, **astringent** is a drying feeling in your mouth as if all of the saliva had evaporated. It is in pomegranates, unripe bananas, some beans, and some leafy greens, such as Swiss chard and spinach.

The sweet taste is heavy and cooling in nature and builds up the tissues of the body. The sour taste is heavy,

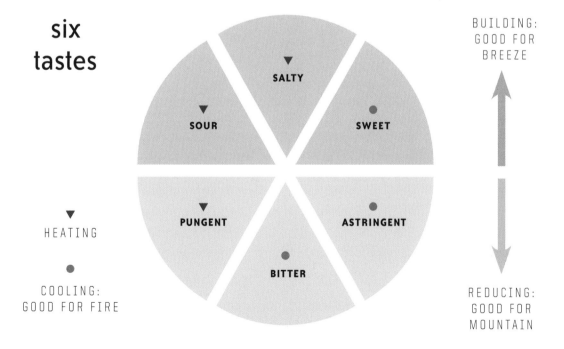

six
tastes

SALTY

SOUR

SWEET

PUNGENT

ASTRINGENT

BITTER

BUILDING:
GOOD FOR
BREEZE

HEATING

COOLING:
GOOD FOR FIRE

REDUCING:
GOOD FOR
MOUNTAIN

moist, and heating in nature, but also builds up the tissues and adds bulk to the body. The salty taste is heating and helps to hold moisture in the body, so it also aids in creating more bulk by retaining water. The pungent taste is strongly heating, and this helps to create movement, melts cold accumulations, and burns up waste products. Bitter and astringent tastes, which are both light and cooling, aid the body in breaking down accumulations and tissues. Astringent reduces moisture. In a nutshell, sweet, sour, and salty tastes build tissues, and pungent, bitter, and astringent tastes break down tissues. We all need both building and breaking down to happen every day as old cells constantly break down (catabolic activity) and must be replaced by new ones (anabolic activity). Nevertheless, certain individuals need more of one action and less of the other.

discerning the six tastes

Even though your body instinctively knows what to do with each taste, that does not mean that your mind necessarily understands the tastes and can discern them. It may take time to train your mind to understand and distinguish each taste. I suggest saying the word aloud as you taste it, to develop a strong association.

The sweet, sour, and salty tastes may be the easiest for you to discern if the bulk of your diet consists of fast foods, packaged foods, and processed foods, which rely heavily on these three tastes. Bitter and astringent are the tastes that are commonly lacking in our modern diet. Tasting bitter greens, green tea, or a bitter gourd (a green, bumpy vegetable sold in Indian markets, shown on page 5) will help you to make the connection between mind and tongue. Bitter and astringent tastes are often together in foods, particularly in foods we consider medicinal herbs, so it may be hard to separate them at first. Use a green unripe banana to discover the astringent taste alone without an excessively bitter taste.

food basics for breeze types

The light, cold, and dry Breeze individuals, who need more mass, insulation, and moisture, will benefit from eating more foods that are sweet, sour, and salty. These tastes give their bodies the adequate building blocks to create more muscle, store more adipose (fat) tissue, and retain more water.

Ideal foods for the Breeze type are warm—both in temperature and nature—moist, oily, nourishing, and well cooked. Cooking is a way of predigesting foods to increase the chances of proper digestion and make the nutrients more bioavailable. This is helpful for the often delicate and always variable digestive fire of the Breeze. Heavier foods like proteins, dairy, fats, and whole grains are all good for an individual with this constitution, to build healthy muscle and fat stores for strength and insulation. This is particularly true if the choices are also warming in nature, to counter the cold quality that predominates in the Breeze individual.

Chicken, turkey, eggs, or beef, in addition to easily digested legumes like mung beans, are good choices of protein. All dairy is good, particularly yogurt, buttermilk, or kefir, because these are warming in nature due to fermentation. A proper amount of healthy fat is essential in the form of warming oils, animal fats, or ghee. The best whole grain choices are basmati rice, brown rice, or oats. Vegetables and fruits should be well cooked, because raw foods can be hard for a weak digestive fire to process fully. If you are vegetarian or vegan, you can easily find heavy, naturally sweet grains, vegetables, nuts, and beans that can nourish you as well as meat or dairy can. The best vegetables for Breeze individuals are heavy, sweet, and warming, such as root vegetables—specifically carrots, beets, and yams. Sweet, juicy fruits such as berries, mangoes, cherries, and bananas are ideal. For a complete list of "Eat More" foods, see page 100. It is important to keep in mind that even though dense, heavy, naturally sweet foods like dairy and

TASTE AND ACTION IN THE BODY

Taste is the first signal to the body to start digestion. The tongue tastes a particular flavor and then the body knows which acids or enzymes to produce to properly digest the coming food. Taste is also a clue about the action or effect the food will create in the body when digested (called the post-digestive effect, or *vipaka*). This connection between the taste of food and its action in the body explains why animals know exactly which food is right for them in each climate, season, and stage of life. Animals use their sense of smell and taste to discern which foods would be medicine. To make good decisions, they do not need to know caloric intake, nutritional percentages, or the chemical compositions. Nature has provided us a simpler plan to health, and we, too, can learn to find our own food-medicines.

some meats benefit Breeze individuals, because they have delicate digestive systems, portions should be small.

mountain basics

To stay in balance, the Mountain has markedly different food requirements than the Breeze has. Individuals who already have abundant moisture and a heavy build do not need to eat as many foods from the sweet, sour, and salty categories. Even a moderate amount of heavy, sweet grains; sour, juicy fruits; or salt may cause them to gain weight or swell from excessive water retention. The Mountain needs the three remaining tastes: pungent, bitter, and astringent. Foods with these tastes, particularly vegetables, are lighter and will increase the Mountain's ability to break down old tissues and remove excess fluids.

Foods that are warm, dry, light, rough, spicy, and heating in nature are best for this type. Cooking foods also aids the Mountain types in proper digestion, because they often have a cool, dull, or slow digestive fire. Abundant vegetables are required for the bulk of their diet if this type is to remain healthy. Many vegetables are light in nature and

packed with nutrients, minerals, phytochemicals, and energy, so the Mountain can meet most nutritional requirements by eating a wide variety of vegetables. They need limited grains, fats, and protein in their diet, to prevent excess heaviness, weight gain, or fluid retention. Avoiding or limiting all dairy, animal products, and most sweeteners is best for their health. Fruits are better for the Mountain when dried.

Light grains such as millet, amaranth, and corn are good choices. Plant-based proteins are lighter, with less fat; legumes, fermented soy products such as tempeh, or light seeds such as pumpkin and sunflower are healthy options. All vegetables are good except the sweet, juicy, or slimy ones, for example, sweet potato, cucumbers, or okra, respectively, and it is usually better to eat them cooked rather than raw. In moderation, dried apricots, cranberries, figs, and raisins are good fruits for the Mountain. Only honey or minimally processed or homegrown stevia (see page 38) should be used as sweeteners—and in small amounts. The Mountain type should use oils sparingly. For a complete list of "Eat More" foods, see page 133.

STEVIA: TO USE OR NOT TO USE?

Stevia is a plant that has a naturally sweet flavor and a slightly bitter aftertaste. The sweetness is thirty to forty times that of raw sugar, so only a small amount is required. It is increasing in popularity and sold as a natural, healthy alternative to sugar, but the highly processed forms of stevia flooding the market are far from natural or healthy. Most are processed with chemicals to remove the aftertaste or to change the natural color from green to white. They may also contain other forms of sugars. To ensure that your stevia is the real thing, you can make your own. It is simple, easy, and inexpensive. Check out wholelifestylenutrition.com for instructions.

fire basics

The Fire type needs the three tastes that are cooling in nature—sweet, bitter, and astringent—for the bulk of their diet. The cooling nature of these flavors balances the natural heat of the Fire type.

A strong appetite and sharp digestive fire encourage Fire individuals to eat heartily. It is important that they eat enough heavy, nourishing foods that they can make it from one meal to the next without becoming *hangry*—the angry, irritable feeling that arises in a Fire individual when her previous meal has been digested and the strong digestive juices in her stomach are now beginning to eat away at her, potentially triggering her to lash out at anyone or anything that adds even the slightest amount of irritation to her mounting hunger. (Although *hangry* may not be in the dictionary, many people relate to the feeling.) The entire nervous system can be agitated when the Fire individual does not eat enough food, and heat will rise, physically and emotionally, creating more Fire imbalance. This makes cooling foods that nourish and sustain important staples for the Fire types.

A diet consisting mostly of cooling fruits, vegetable, grains, legumes, or animal proteins (if you consume them) nuts, seeds, sweeteners, and minimal amounts of fats or oils typically serves a Fire individual well. Fruits that are juicy and cooling include avocadoes, apples, melons, grapes, pears, and figs. Green vegetables such as leafy greens, broccoli, zucchini, peas, green beans, and cucumbers are the most cooling. Nourishing grains include basmati rice, oats, wheat, and barley. All legumes are good protein options, as are cooling nuts and seeds such as coconut, almond, pumpkin, and sunflower. Sweet dairy such as milk and ghee are more cooling than fermented forms are. If you eat meat, chicken, turkey, and venison are the best options for the Fire individual, and you can use coconut, sunflower, safflower, and olive oils regularly in moderation. Raw foods are often appropriate for Fire individuals, because their sharp digestive fire can often handle the rough, cold, and hard qualities of those foods. For a complete list of "Eat More" foods, see page 163.

SPICE-MEDICINES

Spices are concentrated food-medicines that display the six tastes in a stronger form than most foods do. Relative to other foods, only a small amount of a spice is required to have an effect on the tongue or the body. Cinnamon is sweet, pungent, bitter, and astringent in taste, and it makes a delicious condiment for sweet grains or cooked fruits. However, if you try to eat a spoonful, you may start to choke due to the strong astringent quality that dries up the secretions in your mouth and throat upon contact. Drawing on cinnamon's astringency, you could use it to dry up the excess secretions produced during a cold by making a tea and drinking it frequently. Regular consumption of cinnamon in foods and drinks could be a preventive measure for Mountain types, to reduce accumulation of mucus. Conversely, a dry Breeze individual might try to limit use of this spice to ensure that adequate moisture remains in the body for lubrication.

Before the modern convenience of refrigeration, humans relied on spices for their preservative qualities as well as for their digestive and health-enhancing properties. Spices that healed wounds, prevented illness, and eased discomforts were a part of the home apothecary. People used ginger in steam to clear the sinuses of mucus or applied it to the body as a poultice, to ease stiffness of muscles and joints. They used cardamom, cinnamon, black pepper, and garlic internally to prevent colds and flus, and coriander tea as a wash for the eyes, to reduce inflammation. Turmeric acted as a natural antibiotic. Nutmeg with its astringent qualities could stop diarrhea.

Ayurveda still regards the kitchen as the medicine cabinet. Spices certainly can make food more delicious, but individual spices used at the right times by the right individual can also be medicinal. As with food, individuals should choose a spice based on their constitution, their imbalance, or the season to benefit from the spice's health-enhancing effects.

In general, to stimulate appetite, improve digestion, warm the body, dispel gas or bloating, and improve circulation, Breeze individuals do well with sweet, warming spices that are not overly heating. Ginger, hing, cardamom, and tulsi, also known as holy basil, are good examples. Keep in mind that spices that are too heating can dry the tissues, so although the warmth of some spices is good for Breeze types, they should avoid eating an excessive amount of hot, spicy foods. The Mountain, on the other hand, may do well with strong, hot, stimulating spices that build heat, create movement, dry up accumulations, and dispel stagnation— spices such as black pepper, paprika, garlic, cinnamon, and ginger. The Fire needs spices that can improve digestion (without adding excess heat), reduce inflammation, and cool the mind and heart, such as coriander, cumin, fennel, turmeric, and rose. The "Eat More" lists in chapters 8 through 10 can help you understand which foods, tastes, and spices to choose regularly for better health. Spices appropriate for your type also make your food easier to digest, and Ayurveda regards this as extremely important.

sharp digestive fire

Just because the Fire type enjoys a sharp digestive fire, that may not always be healthy. If the liquid component of pitta increases too much, this can weaken a person's digestive power and lead to loose stools. If you find you cannot miss a meal, you need to eat, but you have loose stools, ulcers, or gastritis and are not digesting your food well, you may want to consult with your personal health care practitioner for more tailored recommendations.

—DR. CLAUDIA WELCH

"When diet is proper, medicine is not needed.
When diet is improper, medicine will not work."

—Translation from *Charaka Samhita*, an ancient Ayurvedic textbook

CHAPTER FOUR

healthy eating guidelines

ACCORDING TO RISHIS, the wise seers of Ayurveda, the human being is composed of many layers or sheaths, called *koshas*. The layers are systematically arranged from the gross physical components to subtler and more expansive layers. Three koshas are applicable for our purposes: the physical body, the energetic body, and the mental body. The physical form of our bodies is the first layer, called the "food body," because we rely on food to build and maintain every cell of our being. The second layer is the electromagnetic field that permeates our physical body and extends beyond the boundaries of our skin to surround us, also called the "energy" or "prana body." The third is the "mental body," which is the matrix of our thoughts, feelings, perceptions, and emotions and permeates both the physical and prana bodies.

To become a balanced and vibrant person, one must attend to nourishment of the food body, so that all of the other bodies have a strong and stable root. We are nourished by wholesome quality foods, fresh pure water, and oxygen, but also, just as importantly, by the senses, nature, our relationships, and our spiritual practices. Infants given adequate nutrition but deprived of touch will not thrive. That speaks loudly to what is truly important for a human being. Ayurveda considers all of these things important.

definition of prana

Prana is the vital life force that exists in us and around us. It is the energy that animates all life or that causes a seed to grow. It is also the flow of intelligence, or awareness, that allows all parts of the body to communicate and work harmoniously together.

NOURISHING THE "FOOD BODY"

Because food creates every cell of the body, the quality of the food we ingest is extremely important. Chemicals, pesticides, hormones, antibiotics, and artificial colorings and flavorings are not food and confuse the intelligence of the body, because we do not make use of these substances as nourishment. Foods that have been highly processed have little remaining energy and, therefore, offer the body little nourishment or none at all. These nonfood substances can be toxic to the body and must be eliminated by the hard work of the liver, kidneys, and other organs of elimination. If we eat contaminants regularly, these organs may become overworked or overwhelmed and the body will store toxins that should have been eliminated. To avoid toxic accumulations and to nourish the "food body," follow a few basic guidelines.

food basics

Food is a gift from nature. When it comes to making healthy choices, simplicity is best. Fresh fruits and vegetables recently harvested still have their life force (prana) intact, and this means more energy for you. A seed, nut, legume, or grain can be planted in the earth and sprout life—that is life force! Whole foods are the staples that make delicious and nutritious meals and contribute to good health. Ayurveda considers everything to be potential food-medicine, including animal products and dairy when used by the right person at the right time—and provided that you choose to eat them. Ayurveda helps us get what we need, whether we are vegetarian or not. If you do eat animal products, they should be in their natural state, free from contaminants, and without excessive processing.

Modern society inundates us with unhealthy foods. Ninety percent of the products at any given grocery store are packaged, processed, or filled with contaminants. It is difficult to go even one day without seeing advertising for these products. On top of that, our social world revolves around food, and the food provided to you at a gathering may not be what you would choose for yourself. These are obstacles to eating well. Try to make healthier choices whenever possible and give yourself a pat on the back when you do this more often.

One criterion that helps us categorize foods as healthy or unhealthy is whether we can digest those foods well. If we can digest them well, they serve to nourish our tissues. If we cannot, they have a negative effect on our tissues. What one person can digest easily may be difficult for another to digest. One man's meat is another man's poison. We will go into greater detail later, but here is a general list of foods that are most likely to support healthy digestion.

Choose:

- ∻ Organic, locally grown fruits, vegetables, nuts, seeds, legumes, and whole grains;
- ∻ Organic, cold-pressed oils extracted without the use of chemicals;
- ∻ Raw, organic, and whole dairy products, if you eat them;

❖ Organic animal products produced without the use of growth hormones, antibiotics, steroids, or feed grown with toxic chemicals or pesticides, if you eat them;

❖ Organic and natural spices and herbs (for example, use naturally harvested sea or mineral salt instead of iodized, refined table salt);

❖ Organic, 100% fruit and vegetable juices, not from concentrate;

❖ Natural sweeteners like raw honey, raw sugar, whole cane sugar, maple syrup, or minimally processed or homegrown stevia;

❖ Organic herbal teas; and

❖ Foods that have not been genetically modified or engineered.

The following are foods that will likely hinder digestion, so aspire to reduce or eliminate your intake of the following:

❖ White flour and refined white sugar;

❖ Caffeine and other stimulants;

❖ Excessive alcohol;

❖ Processed foods—frozen, canned, packaged, or fast foods;

❖ Hydrogenated oils;

❖ Foods with monosodium glutamate (MSG);

❖ Artificial colorings, flavorings, and sweeteners;

❖ *Seafood—limit due to high mercury content, heavy metals, PCBs, DDT, and other pollutants in our oceans;

❖ Cold or carbonated drinks;

❖ Cold and raw foods, except in the appropriate seasons and climate;

❖ Deep-fried foods; and

❖ Red meat, except in small quantities.

water basics

Water brings cohesion and lubrication to the body and is responsible for flushing out waste products. Foods with high water content, such as fresh fruits and vegetables, already have the appropriate amount of water for digestion and assimilation. Foods that have low water content, however, like most packaged and processed foods, are drying and dehydrating. Without adequate hydration, the processes of digestion, assimilation, and elimination may be compromised. In fact, water is essential for most bodily processes, even the relaying of information across synaptic space in the nervous system. So inadequate hydration can have a wide range of negative outcomes, from low energy to improper elimination of wastes, and even lack of focus. A regular lack of water means that wastes will not move out of the body in a timely manner.

Fresh, pure water is an important ingredient for health. Our bodies, like the earth's surface, are composed mostly of water—about 70 percent. We are a microcosm of the macrocosm. If the water on our planet is polluted, guess what? So are we. Very few uncontaminated bodies of water are left on our planet. Ice samples from Antarctica have been found to contain DDT. Obviously, no one was spraying DDT on orange crops in Antarctica as a pesticide, so that means that through the cycling and recycling of water and air, this highly toxic substance has been carried everywhere on Earth.

Some sources of spring water and well water are still free from contaminants. If you have a well, it is a good idea to have the water tested, especially if you live in an area that has a history of mining, oil production, fracking, farming, or other industry. Filtering your water is also a good idea, although many filters are more for taste than health, so be sure to research what your filter does. Ask your water provider or utility company for a water quality report that lists the contaminants found in your water source, and use that information to choose a filter. Water can also pick up toxic heavy metals such as lead from pipes after leaving a water treatment plant, so look into a filter for these as well as bacteria, viruses, volatile organic compounds, and chlorine. Tap water has chlorine, and if that is your main source of water and you do not filter it, leave your drinking water in an open container overnight, so that most of the chlorine can evaporate. If you buy bottled water, store it in a cool space—out of the sun or heat—or keep it in glass containers, as water can be contaminated when soft plastics from the bottle leach into it from heat or long storage.

The next natural question is: How much water should I consume each day? Ayurvedic texts provide only simple guidelines for water intake based on one's constitution. From my personal experience, eight glasses of water is a good general guideline, but again, each body is unique. Breeze individuals need the most water to counter their dry tendency (eight 10-ounce glasses: 80 ounces or 2.4 liters daily). Fire individuals will have a moderate need for water (seven glasses: 70 ounces or 2 liters daily). Mountain

individuals typically need less water (six glasses: 60 ounces or 1.8 liters daily). In general, our own natural intelligence can guide how much water we drink, if we truly pay attention to our thirst—although many people mistake the need for water as hunger. Our bodies will naturally need more water if we are in warm, dry climates or environments, or if we are exercising and sweating regularly.

If you consume coffee, black or green tea, other caffeinated beverages, or alcohol, which dehydrate the body, you may need to consume extra water to compensate. One additional ounce of water per ounce of caffeinated or alcoholic beverage is a good estimate. A person who drinks a 12-ounce (0.35 liter) cup of coffee in the morning and two 8-ounce glasses (0.5 liter) of wine in the evening should drink an additional 28 ounces (0.8 liter) of water in a day.

air basics

Oxygen is the nourishment the body requires most frequently—we can survive only a few minutes without it. When we breathe in air, the body takes in this nourishment along with prana (energy) from the environment. Breath helps to regulate the endocrine system, which is the command center for all activities in the body. The lungs consist of a total of five lobes and require full movement of all the lobes to adequately clear out waste products and have sufficient space to take in precious oxygen and prana. Breathing practices or vigorous exercise are recommended daily to foster this clearing. (Breathing exercises for each body-mind type are discussed in chapters 8 to 10.)

The lungs and sinuses can be passageways for pollutants to enter the body. Cleaning products, detergents, air fresheners, and other household products that contain harsh chemicals are not only toxic to the environment but also to your body. Environmentally friendly household products and body products often contain essential oils from plants that exhibit many of the same antibacterial,

water temperature

Ayurveda recommends drinking all liquids, including water, at room temperature or warmer. Cold or iced drinks can diminish the digestive fire or even impair digestion. Warm or hot water, on the other hand, can help the channels of the body to remain open and improve the movement of the lymphatic system for cleansing.

antiviral benefits of the harsh chemical products, but without the risk to your health and to the planet. In fact, many essential oils help bolster the immune system and create a stronger, more balanced body.

You can improve the quality of indoor air by keeping plants that produce oxygen and clean the air of pollutants. We cannot control some factors of air quality, making the ones we can control even more important. To learn more, check out *How to Grow Fresh Air: 50 Houseplants that Purify Your Home or Office* by B. C. Wolverton.

THE IMPORTANCE OF DIGESTIVE FIRE IN TISSUE FORMATION

To nourish the physical body, we need more than just good ingredients; we also need the right amount of fire in the belly to "cook" the food. A strong and balanced digestive fire is responsible for transforming your food first into a liquefied, "food juice," and then into a more refined substance: *rasa*. Rasa is the cooling, nourishing, liquid aspect of all body tissues. It circulates throughout the body, through the plasma, lymph, blood, and other bodily fluids. Every cell and tissue select the precise nutrients they need from this circulating rasa to build and maintain structure and health. Healthy tissues cannot be built from poor-quality rasa. When digestion is strong, rasa is healthy and our tissues are well nourished. This is why Ayurveda considers the digestive fire and digestion to be the most important factors in creating health.

tips for balanced digestive fire

Think of the stomach like a pot of food and the digestive acids and enzymes like the fire of the stove. If the fire is too low (as is common in the Mountain), it cannot sufficiently cook food. If the fire is too hot (as in the Fire), it will burn food. If the fire is variable (as in the Breeze), it may cook some food and only partially cook other food. Any of those challenges results in cellular "building blocks" that will be of poor quality and either excessive or deficient.

rasa

Rasa is a rich word. It means juice, sap, liquid, mercury, essence, elixir, taste, flavor, charm, emotion, and feeling. Healthy rasa yields interest, enthusiasm, love, and appreciation. We can receive flavor from food and from experience. Consider how we feel when we eat something sweet and compare that to how we feel when we are in loving, supportive company. Both experiences nourish us with a sweetness, a sweet rasa that nourishes our minds and emotions as well as our bodies. When we digest our experiences and our food, we are nourished. When we are unable to digest either, the flavor of life is more complicated. When our experiences are positive and digestion is strong, rasa is healthy and we feel enthusiasm for life, devotion, gratitude, vitality, and love.
—DR. CLAUDIA WELCH

One important way to keep the digestive fire strong is to allow enough time for complete digestion before adding any other food to the "cooking pot." This is common sense. Digestion of fruit alone takes about thirty minutes and vegetables a little longer. A simple meal may take three hours to digest, but a complex and heavy meal with meat—the heaviest and hardest protein to digest—as well as grains and fats, might take up to six hours. The ideal plan is to eat enough food at one meal to get you to the next meal without snacking. But if you do need to snack, make sure to wait at least three hours after your previous meal and to eat something light enough to digest fully before the next meal. Fruit is ideal for that, because it requires the least amount of time to digest. Just make sure that you consume fruit or fruit juice alone and at least thirty minutes before any other food, because their sugars can ferment in the stomach when combined with other foods, slowing or limiting proper digestion.

Water intake is another consideration in keeping the digestive fire strong. A large amount of water consumed right before or with a meal can dilute the digestive juices and weaken the body's ability to process the food. You can consume a small amount of room-temperature or warm water with a meal, but otherwise drink water one hour before a meal or several hours afterward. See the "Daily Schedule" in chapters 8 to 10 for a sample timetable for drinking.

To preserve your digestive fire, focus on chewing your food thoroughly. The saliva in your mouth contains enzymes, which start the process of digestion, mixing with the food as you chew. The teeth macerate and the saliva softens the food until it becomes a liquid. If the food is still in large or hard pieces when swallowed, the digestive fire in the stomach has a much bigger job. Chew each bite thirty to forty times to lessen the load on your digestive system and keep the digestive fire balanced. Take your time, eat slowly, don't rush, and take a deep breath between bites and after finishing your meal.

Eat your meals at regular times every day. A regular schedule will help create stability and routine. Your internal fire will have enough time to build between meals and you will avoid inflaming or putting out your fire by going too long between meals. Regularity will also keep your nervous system relaxed, and this, in turn, will help keep the fire burning strong.

Finally, give your full attention to meals. Involve all the senses in the pleasure and enjoyment of eating, so that you can be present in the moment and give all of your energy

ATTUNING TO THE CYCLES OF NATURE

The intelligence that is innate in us is also all around us. Nature and her cycles follow an intelligent design that provides balance for all the plants and animals, as well as the Earth. We are also part of nature, and when we attune to the cycles and rhythms present, health and balance come more easily. Why swim upstream against the natural cycles when we can turn around and float our way to balance?

to digestion. Whenever possible, eat in a quiet, peaceful setting. Our nervous systems still function as animals' do, and at any sign of danger our bodies will shut down the digestive process so that they have more energy available to flee or fight. We are not yet so sophisticated that our brain can tell the difference between the stress response we have to a life-threatening encounter and the one we have from imagining a challenging situation at work or seeing violence on the news. To reduce outside stimulation and improve the chance of complete digestion, it is best to avoid distractions like television, computer, and work while eating, and to limit reading or talking while you eat a meal.

In addition to these basic guidelines for improving and preserving a balanced digestive fire, Ayurveda offers important information to complete the picture of healthy eating. It answers the questions of how much to eat, what to eat in each season, and when to eat.

eating with the seasons

In each season, nature provides the foods that will allow us to maintain balance. Examine the seasonal harvest for any geographical area and you will find the food that grows there provides the perfect qualities to ensure that its inhabitants can weather the qualities and effects of the season. The seasons themselves create a system of balance with a season of growth and rest, a season of heat, then cold, and a season of wetness, then dryness.

THE IDEAL QUANTITY OF FOOD

The stomach of a healthy person is approximately the size of his two hands cupped together. Look at your hands and imagine a bowl that fits exactly in your hands—the same size, width, and height as your cupped hands. Now visualize the bowl filled two-thirds full with food—half solid and half liquid. That is your ideal quantity of food for each meal when you are in your optimum state of health. Is that more or less than you usually eat at one meal?

Ayurveda maintains that the stomach reaches its ideal capacity when it is one-third full of solid food, one-third full of liquid foods, and one-third with air or space. When this happens, the body creates a signal, so that you will know it has reached a perfect capacity. A small burp or uprising energy from your stomach is the signal. It might be a silent, bubble-like sensation or a fully audible belch.

Have you ever noticed it? Although this is the signal that the stomach is adequately full, it does not necessarily mean that the mind or the tongue is satiated.

In a state of health, contentment and the burp are linked. We are surrounded by an abundance of food in our modern culture, however—a challenge not many cultures throughout history have had the opportunity to encounter—and our health problems are typically ones of excess. It is easy to eat more than necessary without even realizing that you are doing so. If contentment is your only gauge for proper food intake, you will most likely overeat. The stomach will continue to stretch and accommodate more food when you eat before contentment appears. Instead of waiting for a feeling of contentment, we need to listen to the intelligence that nature provides us.

eat for the season or for your imbalance?

When we are in a relative state of balance, the foods that nature provides in each season will likely help us maintain that balance. Once we have gone out of balance, however, we need to observe a diet that will counter the heightened qualities in us, regardless of season. Following a diet specific for your predominant imbalance will be required for a time until you come back to health. Once imbalance symptoms disappear, follow a seasonal diet while always being aware of your constitutional needs.

The seasons each resemble one of the three doshas. Spring, at least in many locations, is cool and wet, with cloudy, heavy, and rainy days that result in sticky, slimy, and muddy earth—all the qualities associated with the Mountain type or kapha dosha. In summer, the days grow warm, then hot; moisture wanes and the long, bright days are full of activity and movement as the season of growth bursts wide open; this is like the heat and transformation of Fire type or pitta dosha. In autumn, days grow colder, the air is dry, and vegetation dries up, increasing the Breeze qualities or vata dosha. In winter, cold accumulates and, depending on where you are, either dryness accumulates or it is very wet, increasing either Mountain or Breeze qualities. But in either case, we return again to the spring, when the frozen elements of winter melt and begin to flow again.

Spring season starts with tiny green shoots—the first of the year—that are bitter, astringent, or pungent in taste. Foods with these tastes provide a natural cleansing action to remove the accumulated stores from the winter and a heating action that counters the cold moistness from the environment. Eating an abundance of these foods is appropriate for most of us in the spring.

The summer brings more activity and more warmth in which sweet berries and fruits can grow, along with the first of the light summer vegetables, including leafy greens. These foods are sweet, juicy, or cooling in nature and give the body a balance from the accumulating heat of the season while nourishing us in this active time.

Finally, in the late summer and early autumn, the harvest of grains and heavy, dense vegetables brings foods that are more warming and building, to counter the mounting cold. The body uses these heavier foods to store up an extra layer of fat insulation for winter and to counteract the lightness and dryness of the climate. The season of storage is internal and external—we also store up roots and grains to last throughout the season, and then nuts, seeds, beans and—if we eat them—animal products like eggs, fats, and meats to supply what storage cannot. These foods are the most warming and heaviest and help insulate the body from the cold, dry, rough, and depleting nature of nature itself in the winter season. From here the cycle starts again, complete with a natural spring cleanse to clear out all the accumulations from the winter.

This is a beautiful yet simple system. The main challenge is that in our marketplace of abundance that lacks a strong connection to the natural environment, it is often difficult to know what to eat. The supermarkets have a harvest from the world at our fingertips in every season, and the choices change minimally with the seasons.

One way to stay connected with the natural seasonal

harvest is to shop at a co-op that supports local farmers or at a nearby farmers' market. A resurgence in local and seasonal eating as a sustainable and environmentally friendly practice has made fresh, seasonal food more accessible to all—from farm-to-table restaurants to locally grown items highlighted in products, recipes, menus, and markets. Another option is to follow your tongue and choose foods with the appropriate tastes for each season: bitter, astringent and pungent in spring; sweet, bitter, and astringent in summer; and sweet, sour and salty in autumn and altering as necessary in winter.

NATURE'S DAILY CYCLE

The cycle of the seasons can offer information about what to eat, and the cycle of the day can tell us when to eat and when not to eat. The three doshas each predominate in a particular part of the day and night for approximately a four-hour period, and, if we understand this ebb and flow, we can make choices that will optimize our energy.

The sun sets in the evening, the temperature cools overnight, and by morning, moisture in the environment condenses. This is true in the mountains or the desert, in warm weather when you will see dew on the ground, or in cold weather when you will see frost. The cool, moist, and heavy qualities that predominate at this time of the morning are like the kapha dosha (Mountain).

These qualities will have an effect on you. You might feel heavy if you wake late in the morning, and if you fall back to sleep, you feel even heavier then next time you wake. This feeling may be compounded if the weather also has cool, moist, and heavy qualities, as during a rainstorm; you might feel as if you need a crane to lift you out of bed. But by knowing the principle of opposites, you might counter this feeling with movement, exercise, a warm drink, a light and warming diet, or breath practices.

The peak of the sun at noon is also the peak of your digestive fire. The hot, light, and sharp qualities that are like pitta dosha (Fire) predominate at this time of day in both the external environment and your internal environment. It makes sense, then, to use this rising of fire to digest food. In fact, it is the ideal time for your biggest meal, because you have a better chance of complete digestion. It is also advisable to use the principle of opposites to make good choices to cool the body. A vigorous training session for a marathon in the peak of the sun will definitely increase your fire. A gentle walk by a cool lake might be a better choice to keep the fire under control.

cycle of the day

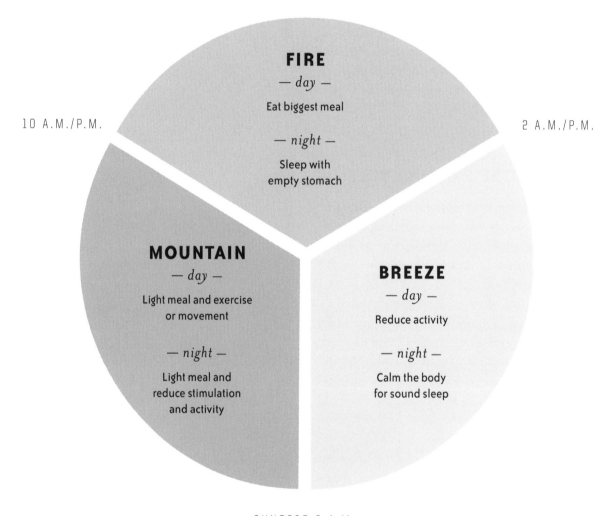

10 A.M./P.M.

2 A.M./P.M.

FIRE

— *day* —

Eat biggest meal

— *night* —

Sleep with
empty stomach

MOUNTAIN

— *day* —

Light meal and exercise
or movement

— *night* —

Light meal and
reduce stimulation
and activity

BREEZE

— *day* —

Reduce activity

— *night* —

Calm the body
for sound sleep

SUNRISE 6 A.M.
SUNSET 6 P.M.

Vata dosha (Breeze) governs the transition times of the day, dusk and dawn, as they are related to change. The qualities of the Breeze, particularly mobility, increase at this time of day. The mind will become active and mobile, so these are good times for meditation. Too much physical mobility at this time of day may drain the reserves and leave you feeling tired. Ayurveda teaches us to eat our final meal early in the evening—so that we go to bed with a light stomach—and to enjoy a light meal, because the digestive fire is naturally lower at this time of day. In this transition time, the doshic cycle starts again.

Now it is important to slow down the body and mind during the second kapha time in preparation for a rejuvenating, sound sleep. Too much stimulation in the evening hours from television, computers, movies, or mental activity can impede this preparation. Calming practices of self-care, meditation, breathing practices, or relaxing yoga poses can help to nudge the body and mind into a restful state.

The second pitta time starts around 10 p.m., with an uprising of heat that can bring hunger again—we often recognize this energy as our "second wind." Once it starts, the fire or second wind does not subside until about 2 a.m. This surge of internal fire is intended to clean out any toxins in the body that have accumulated that day. If the belly is full, the fire will be digesting food, not cleaning the house. This self-maintenance will not be possible if you are not asleep between the hours of 10 p.m. and 2 a.m. It is therefore vital to eat a light meal, early in the evening, so that the belly can be empty before 10 p.m. Once the fire rises, it is difficult for sleep to happen (difficulty falling asleep at this time is likely due to a Fire imbalance). The second wind can be a useful time for creativity, work, or projects, but it comes at the expense of your sleep and therefore your health.

The final vata period of this cycle is in the early morning hours before and encompassing sunrise. The mobility of the mind will predominate if sleep is not sound, creating insomnia. If this happens, use the practices for calming the nervous system in the daily self-care section of chapter 8 to relax and return to sleep. This is the time that yogis and other spiritual seekers traditionally choose to practice meditation, yoga, or chanting, to harness the energy of the mind and counter vata or Breeze imbalances.

During this time of the morning, the mobile quality stimulates the organs of elimination. It is advisable, therefore, to empty or clear the bladder, bowels, lungs, and skin upon rising, so that the body does not reabsorb the toxins eliminated through the self-maintenance of pitta overnight. Daily cleansing practices to clear the senses at this time are also recommended.

Waking around sunrise is advised for everyone, though each body-mind type has different sleep requirements that influence the ideal time. Mountain individuals require only five to six hours of sleep and may feel heavy and lethargic if they sleep more, so waking before sunrise is ideal. Fire individuals need about seven hours of sleep, so they can wake up at sunrise. Breeze individuals require the most sleep, so they can start the day an hour after sunrise.

Daily choices about how much to eat, what to eat, and when to eat, in addition to the basic dietary guidelines for each type, are the foundational building blocks of good health. The body also requires seasonal cleansing to remove toxins accumulated from our food, water, and air, as well as the excess doshas accumulated from the influence of the seasons, inappropriate lifestyle practices, and ignoring the intelligence of the body.

Sweetness of Fall, page 122.

why do we need to cleanse?

ACCORDING TO AYURVEDA, a balanced digestive fire is one of the most important elements responsible for health in the body and, therefore, an imbalanced digestive fire is the first step in creation of disease. As we explored in the previous chapter, an imbalance of Breeze, Fire, or Mountain can lead to disruption of the normal digestive fire and formation of poor-quality tissues. This disruption can also lead to the production of a substance much like glue that can affect the proper functioning of the body. When this happens, cleansing is the only way to restore balance.

UNDERSTANDING THE BUILDUP OF TOXINS

Improperly processed or partially processed food creates a sticky substance that the body cannot use to build healthy tissues, and this substance is difficult to eliminate from the system. The substance is called *ama* in Ayurveda. Ama does not serve a physiological, healthy function in our bodies. On the contrary, it clogs channels, blocks the proper flow of nutrients, and prohibits waste removal, until it finally weakens the ability of your body to do its job. Physical symptoms such as stiff or achy joints, heaviness, lethargy, digestive discomfort, gas, bloating, acid reflux, bad breath, constipation, and diarrhea are all signs of accumulated ama.

Factors in accumulation of ama include poor dietary habits, imbalanced digestive fire, and imbalances or impairment of the natural function in the small intestine, the large intestines, the liver, the pancreas, or the lymphatic system. As we learned in chapter 4, we must also sleep with an empty stomach at the appropriate time of night, so that the body can accomplish the important job of self-cleaning. If wastes are excreted at the proper time of night but the organs of elimination are not cleaned or emptied in the morning, the body may reabsorb these toxins and ama. We must attend to all of these factors to prevent the accumulation of ama.

In addition to faulty eating practices and digestion creating ama, we are almost all exposed to chemical substances, cancer-causing agents, and toxins from the environment. These substances are also ama and are lipophilic, meaning that they attach to lipids, or fats, in the body, and the lymphatic system must detoxify and eliminate them. The lymphatic system is like our internal plumbing for waste removal, but it is also connected to our immune system, so that white blood cells can detoxify wastes and make them innocuous enough for removal through the blood stream and organs of elimination. The body does this job naturally, but many factors (as mentioned above) can impede this process and force the body to store these toxins instead of eliminating them.

The guiding intelligence of the body, knowing that ama will block normal functions of digestion, assimilation, and elimination, will try to store toxins and undigested sludge in a space outside of the digestive tract. Fat, or adipose tissue, is one main site of storage for toxins, to keep them out of circulation. Other spaces in the body that are weakened by trauma, injury, illness, and genetic inheritance, or inherently weak spots, can also become storage sites. Once ama

has been created and stored, we must use cleansing practices that lighten the body.

The classic texts of Ayurveda classify qualities, foods, and practices into two opposing categories. *Langhana*, or lightening, refers to qualities, foods, or actions that lighten the body or create a cleansing action. *Brahmana*, or building, is used to describe nourishing qualities, foods, and actions, employed when rejuvenation is needed. Lightening will remove stored wastes and can invigorate the body, but it will also weaken the body in the process, so building is required to return the tissues to fullness of strength. Each body-mind type is in need of these two actions, but some need more lightening and others more building due to their natural tendencies.

READING THE TONGUE TO UNDERSTAND IMBALANCE

How do you know if you have ama? Very simply, your body tells you each day if the food from the previous day was digested properly. When you rise in the morning, look at your tongue in the mirror. If you see a coating on your tongue, you will know that you have not adequately digested your food. A thin, white coating that does not disguise the underlying color of your tongue is normal. Any other variation of coating is a sign that something needs to change.

Ayurveda and other Eastern systems, such as traditional Chinese medicine, consider the tongue a map of the body. Every feature of the tongue represents an aspect of the constitution or of imbalance. Any excess coating conveys an accumulation of waste products (ama) and a disruption in healthy processes of digestion, assimilation, or elimination. The tongue is the top end of a long, continuous tube that we call the digestive tract, and it acts as a mirror for the internal, or unseen, functioning of the system. The color of its coating can be a tool for understanding what imbalance is predominating in the body. Getting to know the signs of imbalance can lead you toward adjustments in diet and lifestyle to improve digestive function.

As a reminder from previous chapters, the three body-mind types each have a color or colors associated with imbalance. Accumulations anywhere in the body or in the waste products are white in color when influenced by a Mountain imbalance. Yellow or red are the colors associated with Fire imbalance. Dark brown or grayish discoloration is a sign of a Breeze imbalance. These colors are important to reading the body's messages that display themselves on the tongue every day.

For example, a thick yellow coating on the tongue with a bright red tongue base would indicate that the Fire is high. This might guide you, using the principle of langhana, to lighten the diet and, using the principle of opposites, to include more cooling foods with bitter and astringent tastes in your diet for the day. These two actions combined would help to reduce ama and cool the increased excess heat, with any luck restoring balance. It may take one day or several days of these recommended actions, but the tongue will be the guide. Listen to the wisdom of the body and continue these actions until the yellow coating dissipates.

Alternately, if a thick white coating is predominant on the tongue and the base color is pale, a Mountain imbalance and ama are present. We often see this during a cold with congestion. In this case, lightening the diet or fasting to improve the strength of the digestive fire and ingesting strong pungent spices, along with astringent tastes, would burn up the accumulations of ama. A day of spicy, hot ginger and black pepper tea without the intake of food might be enough to clear up the ama—or several days of a light diet composed of pungent, bitter, and astringent foods may be adequate.

Ama is the fertile soil in which the seed of disease can grow. If we ignore the signs of imbalance, then toxins, ama, and excess doshas can accumulate and have an opportunity to spread to other parts of the body. According to Ayurveda, this accumulation marks the beginning stages, or precursors, of disease.

what is your tongue saying?

- Color of the tongue body:
  pink or dark/Breeze;
  bright red/Fire; or pale/Mountain

- Dark or brownish coating:
  ama with Breeze imbalance

- Yellow coating:
  ama with Fire imbalance

- Thick, white coating:
  ama with Mountain imbalance

THE SIX STAGES OF DISEASE

Imbalance follows a logical progression in the body to the point at which disease manifests, and Ayurveda reveals the steps and symptoms along this journey. Each dosha has a natural site—its homesite—in the digestive tract, where it functions healthfully. Accumulation happens here first, bringing with it minor symptoms of imbalance. It then becomes aggravated in the second stage of dis-ease, bringing stronger imbalances. If allowed to continue in its progression, the dosha will enter the third stage: an overflow from the digestive tract into other sites in the body, and will also create imbalance there.

In the fourth stage of dis-ease (spreading), the accumulated doshas and ama move through the body's channels of circulation and look for a weak site—called *khavaigunya*—in various tissues and organs to make their home. There, they begin to alter the normal qualities of those tissues. In the fifth stage of dis-ease, (relocation), the dosha becomes more rooted in its new home and its qualities become more defined and pronounced as signs and symptoms of illness. Finally in the sixth stage (manifestation), the dosha has not only invaded one place, but has also aggravated surrounding organs and tissues, resulting in a substantial disease complete with symptoms and complications.

> "Just as rasa nourishes its fellow tissues, ama is the juice that nourishes disease."
>
> **—Dr. Robert Svoboda, Bachelor of Ayurvedic Medicine and Surgery**

Why wait until disease manifests to listen to the body? Ayurveda gives us the tools to recognize imbalance and stop it before it progresses into disease. One weakness of our modern system of medicine is that we cannot spot most diseases in the precursor stages and, therefore, prevention is limited. What we often call "early detection" is when a disease is already in the fourth or fifth stage. True early detection is when we can identify a disorder in the first or second stage of disease, and disease prevention is when we can prevent progression into further, more serious stages and even guide those stages backward.

CLEANSING BASICS

Just as there is no single diet appropriate for everyone, no one cleanse is right for everyone. The range of cleanses on the market today is wide and varied. One cleanse may have its participants drinking only liquids for forty days while another requires consumption of only animal proteins and vegetables for a week. There are three-day cleanses for the weekend warrior and three-week intensives that require incredible amounts of discipline to complete. Each type of cleanse is appropriate for someone, but without the framework of Ayurveda it can be difficult to understand which one is right for you.

Your current imbalance is the main factor to consider when determining which type of cleanse to undertake. Evaluating your imbalance each time you decide to cleanse is important, because the relative state of balance or imbalance in our bodies is constantly changing with our geography, the climate, and the season, as well as our diet, lifestyle, and stage of life. If you do not have a single predominant imbalance, choose a cleanse based on your constitution with a mindful consideration to the season in which you are cleansing. A cleanse that is right for your type is crucial if you are looking to create better health without more imbalance.

when to cleanse

Ayurveda specifies the junctions between seasons as the ideal time for cleansing, to clear out any accumulation before it can cause problems in the body. With the exception of the extremes of hot and cold in your climate (see sidebar on page 58), any season is permissible. Cleansing one to three times per year is good maintenance, and this is especially true around the season that is most like your predominant type. For example, it is a good idea for everyone to cleanse at the beginning or end of summer, to clear out accumulated heat in the body before it creates a problem. This is especially important for Fire types, because that additional heat on top of their naturally strong fire will create problems if it is held in the body too long. Mountain types have a greater need to clear out the heavy, moist accumulations in the spring, and Breeze types have a stronger need to counter the cold and dry of fall before the winter arrives.

cleansing guidelines for the breeze

In general, cleansing is most challenging for a Breeze type because cleanses are inherently lightening and the qualities of Breeze are light already. The challenge is to employ sufficient grounding techniques to ensure that the Breeze type will not get more aggravated by cleansing. A **grounding cleanse**, which incorporates warm, well-cooked foods that are easy to digest, is perfect for Breeze individuals or those with a Breeze imbalance. This gives their digestive system a break from more-complicated foods and preserves their delicate digestive fire. A fast, or a diet consisting of only liquid foods such as fresh vegetable juice, herbal teas, and sometimes, exclusively water, is too lightening for the Breeze individual. A diet of only raw foods is too cold and difficult for them to digest, plus the large amount of fiber in those raw foods can be rough and abrasive to their sensitive and often dry colons. Breeze individuals might feel unbearably cold, ungrounded, or anxious from those types of cleanses, responses that lead to more imbalance than health.

Too much change, too quickly in diet and lifestyle, can deplete immunity in Breeze types. They are already light, cold, and sensitive by nature, and need a gentle change. Along with incorporating warming foods, it is essential for the Breeze individual to rest more and engage in grounding practices like gentle yoga, warming breath practices, meditation, and warm oil massage during a cleanse, to enable them to complete the process in a safe, supported way. Adequate time away from the stresses of life is also important to the success of any cleanse, as the Breeze imbalance is directly related to the function of the nervous system.

In any season, a short cleanse or mono diet—a simplifying of the diet by eating one type of food—will serve these individuals, but it is especially important to cleanse in the fall before the weather gets too cold. Proper time and focus on rejuvenation is essential, particularly in the fall, so that the tissues and digestive fire have time to rebuild and move into winter with strength. Chapter 8 has more information to help the Breeze address their specific needs.

cleansing guidelines for the mountain

Mountain types need cleansing that reduces the bulk of their body while still keeping the digestive fire burning strong. They have larger stores of muscle and fat, creating a thicker layer of insulation than the other types have, so although all cleanses tend to be a bit lightening, Mountains need an especially **lightening cleanse** to reduce the bulk of the body. In addition, the stable nature of these individuals enables them to remain grounded and maintain their strength during a dramatic shift in diet. Therefore, a cleanse involving fasting on water or vegetable juice could be acceptable for them in certain conditions, as this forces their bodies to burn accumulated fat stores for energy, greatly reducing the amount of body mass.

But the Mountain type still needs enough heat or fire to keep everything moving. Too much cold from consuming only liquids may cause their digestive system to slow down, dramatically impairing the body's ability to remove wastes and toxins. A lightening cleanse with bitter, astringent, and pungent foods may be more effective than a fast alone. These foods stimulate catabolic activity, the breakdown and removal of old cells and accumulations, while keeping the digestive fire burning strong. In addition, vigorous exercise, exposure to the sun, dry sauna, or other forms of heat that induce sweating will greatly increase the lightening aspects of a cleanse.

Springtime cleansing is most important for the Mountain individual or those with a Mountain imbalance. The accumulated stores from winter need to be eliminated early in the spring or else the liquefying process that kapha undergoes as the weather warms will create uncomfortable symptoms, including sinus congestion, lung congestion, runny nose, itchy eyes, sneezing, headaches in the frontal area around the sinuses, heaviness, lethargy, weight gain, and water retention. These individuals can undergo a long and rigorous cleansing process in any season, but it is particularly helpful in the spring. Chapter 9 has more specific information to help the Mountain plan an appropriate cleanse.

cleansing guidelines for the fire

The Fire types need a **cooling cleanse**, with enough food to keep their strong digestive fire satisfied. A Fire's robust appetite must be satiated by food regularly or the excess heat that builds up creates an imbalance. Fasting or eating too little food could create an internal inferno and disrupt the nervous system. The physical and emotional fire that could potentially build up may counter any other health benefits from a cleanse. Raw foods combined with fresh juice may be appropriate in a hot season or climate, but a mono diet of easily digested foods would be better in a cool season or climate.

Cooling practices that are also calming in nature are ideal to include in a cleanse for this type. Gentle and cooling yoga poses and breath work, easy, noncompetitive exercise in or near water, and massage with cooling oils are all good practices to incorporate into a cleanse. In addition, time away from the world of stimulation and activity gives the mind a well-needed rest.

Heat can easily accumulate in cool seasons, when the external cold encourages the body to hold heat internally, and also in hot seasons, when the influence of the external heat has a powerful effect despite adequate self-care. So cleansing at the beginning or end of the warm summer

CONTRAINDICATIONS FOR CLEANSING

Winter in many regions is a season for storage and insulation, and our bodies naturally bulk up in the cooling fall season to insulate against the cold of winter. Cleansing in the winter in a cold climate is not ideal, because the body requires heavy, oily, and warming foods to counter the cold, dry, rough, and depleting qualities present in the season. Classic Ayurvedic textbooks advise traditional cleansing (we will explore the difference between this and modern cleansing) in this season only when it is a health emergency and only if one can avoid the effects of cold during the process. The texts recommend avoiding elimination therapies in the extremes of your climate—both the peak of heat in the summer and during the winter's extreme cold. Cleansing is also not appropriate for pregnant women, nursing mothers, young children, women during their menses, or anyone in a weakened condition from illness or trauma.

season—or both—is beneficial for the Fire types or those with a Fire imbalance. Chapter 10 has more specific information to help the Fire individual determine the unique combination of elements to incorporate into a cleanse.

cleansing with the cycle of the seasons

A healthy individual with no regular tongue coating and only occasional symptoms of imbalance could use three different cleanses seasonally to maintain health. A grounding cleanse will gently clear the body of accumulations in the fall while maintaining immunity, warmth, and strength for the coming winter. A lightening cleanse is great for spring when the extra insulation from winter needs to be lifted. A cooling cleanse is ideal to counter the heat of summer. This framework of understanding from Ayurvedic wisdom can help make sense of the enormous amount of conflicting information available today about diet, nutrition, and cleansing. Each individual cleanse or style of eating is good for someone, but knowing which one will work for you takes a little deeper knowledge of yourself.

the categories of cleansing

Traditional Ayurvedic cleansing is a practice of lightening the body, so that it can eliminate internal accumulations of toxins from the environment, ama from undigested foods, and excess doshas. This systematic cleansing and rejuvenation is called *panchakarma*. Cleansing steps include cleaning or clearing the digestive tract by strengthening the digestive fire and reducing ama, then oleating, or softening with oil applications, the body internally and externally so that it can remove the excess doshas and toxins from deeper storage through elimination therapies (see chapter 11 for more details). Most cleansing practices or packages available on the market either (a) lighten the body by reducing bulk in the diet; or (b) clear and clean the digestive tract, which is the first, but not the only step

of traditional Ayurvedic cleansing. Most of these modern cleanses, however, do not address the accumulation of doshas.

Since all of these processes come under the term *cleansing*, it is important to differentiate between discrete categories. The first cleansing category involves processes that assist the body in its natural daily cleansing. These include sound sleep at the appropriate time of night, and potentially a massage, healing therapy, or daily practice (like the simple daily routine of cleansing, *dinacharya*, on page 68) that moves the lymphatic system or opens the channels, as well as appropriate diet for your type and season, to pacify the doshas and prevent further production of ama. We will call these **daily cleansing** practices.

The second category relates to lightening practices, which for our purposes have three subcategories. The first is **dietary cleansing** and is defined as changing the diet to include lighter food choices. Many modern cleanses fall under this category. Eating a vegetarian or vegan diet could be a simple example for those in the practice of eating meat, dairy, or other animal products. For someone accustomed to a vegan or vegetarian diet, dietary cleansing could happen by choosing a mono diet of exclusively fruit, exclusively vegetables, or kitchari (the main mono diet used in Ayurveda). These dietary cleansing practices may or may not clear and clean the digestive tract.

We will refer to those lightening practices that improve the digestive fire and burn up ama as **digestive cleansing**. Examples of this include a fast or a mono diet (but only if it is appropriate for your imbalance and accomplishes those two aims). For example, a fast from food while consuming only strongly heating herbal teas would be an appropriate digestive cleanse for a Mountain. But a fast of only cold, moist fruit or vegetable juices could dampen the dull digestive fire of a Mountain and create more ama, even though this diet is lightening in nature; this would be considered a dietary cleanse, but not a digestive cleanse.

group cleansing

Cleansing is a wonderful practice to do in community. It is helpful to have others supporting you, preparing food with you, enjoying meals with you, and sharing the goal of better health—and maybe even bliss. I highly recommend finding friends or family members to join you in the experience of cleansing, so that you can share stories and inspirations along the journey. This is how Ayurveda has been passed along for centuries as the wisdom of life.

If a cleanse can address the diverse needs of different body-mind types, then it is safe to do in groups. Many cleanses, including the 31-day protocol in Part II, involve digestive cleansing, which is safe for most people as long as it is done for a proper duration according to your type. Digestive cleansing is very different from a cleanse to remove the doshas from the deeper tissues of the body, panchakarma. The latter requires deeper knowledge of the client and a clinical assessment to make the cleanse safe and effective. Reserve deeper cleansing practices such as panchakarma for private work with a professional on a one-to-one basis.

In an Ayurvedic mono diet of kitchari (see page 79), the whole digestive system gets a break from more complex or difficult-to-digest foods while consumption of herbal teas balances the digestive fire to address ama. The first stage of panchakarma, translated as *ama burning*, is another example of digestive cleansing during which an Ayurvedic practitioner would recommend specific dietary and herbal changes to clear up ama (see chapter 11).

The final category relates to lightening practices that help remove excess doshas and toxins from storage and is specific to Ayurveda. This includes the oleation and elimination phases of panchakarma. This is different from pacifying the doshas. In daily life, appropriate diet and life-style practices can calm any excessive doshas and reduce symptoms of imbalance, but at some point (after pacifying), it is advisable to remove the old accumulations from storage. This is equivalent to pulling up the roots of disease as opposed to just trimming the plants that sprout from imbalance. All the recommendations from the classic Ayurvedic texts refer to this type of cleansing, which we will call **eliminatory cleansing**, which refers to the use of elimination therapies of panchakarma (see chapter 11).

Another difference between traditional Ayurvedic cleansing and modern cleansing is the focus on preliminary practices before cleansing and rejuvenation practices after cleansing. Ayurveda would recommend a cleanse only after appropriate dietary and lifestyle habits have been established, so that the doshas will be pacified or calmed. A cleanse would also be followed by a period of rejuvenation in which proper diet and self-care practices would have the utmost importance, to restore strength to the body before returning to a "normal" daily routine and diet. These preliminary practices and rejuvenating steps are just as important as the cleansing time itself; otherwise, the health of the body may be diminished instead of improved. All too often cleansing ends abruptly without a plan for reintegrating into one's normal diet and routine.

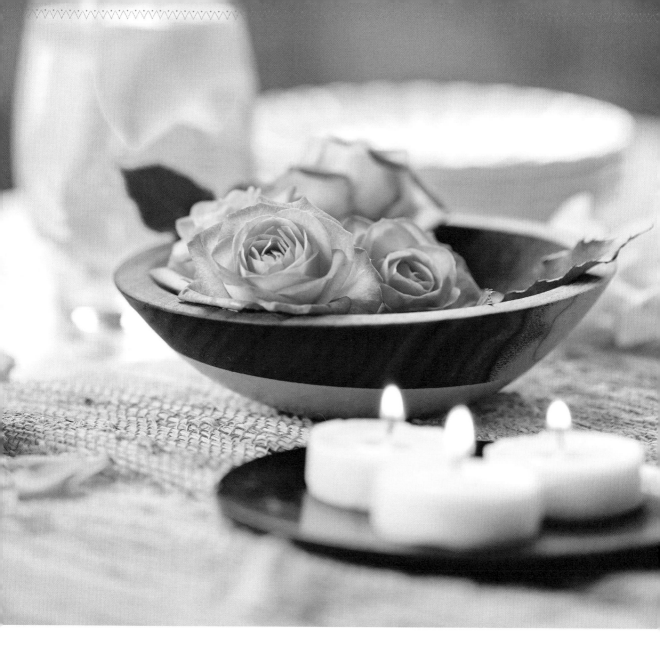

Inappropriate diet or practices at this time when the body is vulnerable can potentially be damaging.

Part II of this book incorporates these preparation and rejuvenation practices, as well as daily cleansing, dietary cleansing, and digestive cleansing practices, into a 31-day protocol for better health. Each one of us is unique and we need to determine which type of cleanse and how much lightening is appropriate for our imbalance, constitution, or both. By applying the knowledge of Ayurveda presented in Part I of this book, we can move on to choosing a cleanse that lightens in just the right amount while maintaining or regaining balance.

cleansing for your body-mind type

tHE RECIPES, lifestyle changes, and self-care practices from this book combine to prepare the body, help bring about a gentle Ayurvedic cleanse, and safely transition back to daily living. These practices make up a 31-day protocol that is explained in chapter 6, but they can always be used for everyday living. After a cleanse, slowly move back to your normal diet and schedule while maintaining the practices you find create the most balance.

If you engage in seasonal cleansing regularly, you may notice that the differences between your "normal" and "cleansing" routines lessen over time. When that happens, you will be ready to engage in more traditional Ayurvedic cleansing (see chapter 11). At that point, the 31-day protocol, which balances the doshas and removes ama and toxins from the digestive tract, will become the preliminary practices to prepare you for eliminatory cleansing that removes deeply rooted excess doshas.

simple eating for everyone

tHIS CHAPTER PROVIDES A 31-DAY protocol that is simple, gentle, and safe for almost everyone. It is designed to create more awareness about food choices and help you to listen to the wisdom of your own body. However, if you have specific health concerns, please consult your physician or health care practitioner to determine whether this diet and the cleanses in this book are right for you.

The first three weeks of the protocol incorporate daily cleansing practices and are the same for everyone, with minimal changes to the diet. The focus, instead, is applying the knowledge of Ayurveda to determine how much to eat, where to eat, and when to eat. These three weeks will give you the foundations for lifelong healthy eating practices.

The fourth week includes dietary cleansing practices that you will choose specifically for your imbalance (or constitution, if there is no predominant imbalance). It will lay out a plan complete with diet and lifestyle recommendations for creating balance. The final three days are the digestive cleansing days, with a limited diet and limited activity. The final segment of this chapter, Transition Time, will also give you suggestions for easing out of the cleanse in a safe and timely manner.

WEEK 1
— finding balance with portion size —

The first week requires no change to your diet, but instead focuses on discovering the right amount of food for each meal. To start, find a bowl that fits perfectly in your two hands and holds the same amount as your two hands cupped together. Fill the bowl only two-thirds full, as the stomach should ideally be one-third full of solid food, one-third full of liquid foods, and one-third with space. Use this bowl when you are eating at home, so that you have a good visual estimate of the proper amount of food.

During meals, give special attention to listening for your burp (see page 47). It may not be audible, but at the very least you will feel a small bubble-like upward movement. It may surprise you to see how early the burp arrives. Once it happens, notice if you feel content or satiated with this amount of food. If not, count the number of bites it takes after the burp to find contentment.

This is your only practice for the week, so try to give it your full attention at every meal. As the week progresses, notice any changes to your awareness. Are you able to recognize the burp at each meal or do you still miss it? Can you predict when the burp will arrive, based on the amount of food you consumed? Are you closer to contentment when it arrives? If the answer is no, observe yourself at meals. Is anything distracting you—conversations, work, television, or something else?

WEEK 2
— mindful eating:
what are you feeding yourself? —

This week, you will shift your attention to the manner and setting in which you eat, as well as the overall quality of the food you consume. You will begin to eliminate stimulating foods from your diet and start consuming more calming foods. The question to ask is, "What am I feeding myself?" The answer may be more complex than you think.

Once you have knowledge of Ayurveda, it is easy to see that the twenty qualities are in and around us at every moment. Our emotions, thoughts, sensory perceptions, conversations, environment, food, and the seasons all affect us. At mealtimes, other qualities are "ingested" along with our food. The question to ask is, "Can I also 'digest' these qualities?" When it comes to emotions, those such as grief, sadness, anger, or fear can completely stamp out the digestive fire. For this reason Ayurveda recommends eating only when emotions are calm and stable.

On a more subtle level, this concept is true for all of the components present during a meal. A busy, loud, and stimulating environment may affect the nervous system and decrease the strength of the digestive fire. An uncomfortably hot, moist setting or season can inflame or impair the appetite. A stimulating conversation, television program, or book can divert digestive energy away from the belly to the mind, slowing digestion. We must have enough power to digest our food as well as the qualities we are "feeding" ourselves during each meal.

In Ayurveda, three categories classify the basic energetics, the action or essence predominant in a substance or activity, of the mind, food, and activities—calming, stimulating, or dulling. Foods that are calming in nature (*sattvic*, or the natural state of the mind) create a sense of stillness, peace, clarity, purity, and contentment. Foods that are stimulating in nature (*rajasic*) create movement and heat, bringing with them cravings, irritations, and desire for more stimulation. Dulling foods (*tamasic*) create inertia of body and mind with heavy, cloudy, and lethargic sensations.

The qualities of foods, environment, and mind affect digestion. For example, a quiet, peaceful environment for meals can create a calm state of mind; a violent television program or emotions of anger can create a heated, stimulated state of mind; and news of a tragic event can trigger a heavy, dull state of mind. Eating calming foods in a calming setting with calm emotions will have the result of a calm body and mind: This is the goal.

Look at the lists that follow and notice whether the foods you consume regularly are calming, stimulating, or dulling. This week, start to eliminate the stimulating and dulling foods, so that by the end of it you are eating mostly calming foods. Eliminate alcohol, coffee, caffeinated foods or beverages, carbonated drinks, processed white sugar and flour, packaged, canned, and fast foods, deep-fried foods, and red meat for the remainder of the month. Try to eat freshly prepared foods whenever possible, particularly those you make yourself.

Notice the environment in which you eat regularly. What other qualities are you feeding yourself? Start to shift your habits by eating in a quiet and calm environment, avoiding television, work, computers, or reading during a meal, and limiting conversations. Take time to focus on the process of digestion and your enjoyment of the tastes, textures, colors, and aromas of your food. Use all your senses, and chew slowly and thoroughly. Continue to listen for your burp and be aware of contentment when it arises.

Energetics of Food

Calming foods are naturally sweet and building in nature. They include the following:

+ fresh fruits and vegetables (except heating ones)
+ whole grains, particularly rice, wheat, quinoa, and oats
+ beans (in moderation), especially mung, aduki, or soy/tofu
+ raw soaked nuts and seeds of almonds, sesame seeds, cashews, and coconut
+ raw and/or organic dairy products from cows or goats that have been treated well, especially milk, ghee, soft cheese, or fresh homemade yogurt
+ natural sweeteners, such as raw sugar, raw honey, maple syrup, and jaggery
+ moderate amounts of sweet spices such as ginger, cardamom, cinnamon, fennel, cumin, coriander, and saffron
+ garden herbs, such as mint, basil, cilantro, and tulsi
+ food prepared with love and awareness

Stimulating foods are highly seasoned, heating in nature, and create movement. They include the following:

+ coffee, caffeinated beverages, and chocolate
+ carbonated drinks
+ heating and sour fruits, such as sour oranges, guava, tamarind, and pineapple
+ heating vegetables, such as radishes, eggplant, garlic, peppers, and onions
+ millet and corn
+ nuts (except almonds, cashews, coconut, peanuts, or rancid nuts)
+ dairy products that are sour, such as sour cream or buttermilk
+ seafood and chicken
+ heating spices such as black pepper, chili pepper, paprika, and curry
+ heating garden herbs, such as rosemary, thyme, oregano, and chives
+ refined, artificial, or highly processed sweeteners

Dulling foods are heavy, lacking prana (energy), stale, partially cooked, overcooked, fruits that are overripe or under ripe, and processed sweets or overly processed foods in general. They include the following:

+ alcohol
+ garlic, onions, and mushrooms
+ processed, refined, and bleached flour of grains
+ wheat

- urad dal (legume)
- peanuts and rancid nuts
- hard cheese and highly processed dairy products
- red meats
- nutmeg and jalepeño
- molasses and highly-processed stevia
- canned, frozen, or highly processed foods

Note: Mountain individuals need some stimulating foods to create internal heat and movement, and Breeze individuals can also tolerate a small amount. Unless living a life of seclusion or meditation and contemplation, the Fire and Breeze types usually require some amount of heavy and dulling foods to build strength and keep them heavy enough to do their work in the world and sleep soundly.

WEEK 3
— attuning to the cycle of the day —

Now you will shift your attention to eating at the proper times of day, drinking a proper amount of water for your type at appropriate times, and developing rituals for mealtimes, mornings, and evenings. This will bring you stability, ensure better digestion and elimination, and establish basic self-care practices you will expand in week 4.

Review the cycle of the day from chapter 4 (pages 49 to 51) and notice ways you can adjust your schedule to accommodate these recommendations. Start with meals: Eat your largest or heaviest meal at noon, eat lighter meals in the morning and evening, and eat at established and regular times every day. Find ways to make your meals feel like a sacred ritual: Light a candle, express gratitude for the food, take a few deep breaths and calm yourself before eating, or have a special cup of tea before or after meals. Continue to use all the practices from weeks 1 and 2 at every meal.

Review the section on water intake (page 44) and determine the proper amount you need. Make a plan to incorporate water breaks in the day so that you consume an adequate amount without impeding digestion: Drink one hour before or two hours after a meal (see the daily schedule in chapters 8 to 10 for a sample plan). Start with a large glass of warm water upon rising and then carry a glass or stainless steel water bottle with you throughout the day, so that you can drink when you are thirsty. Water is essential for the cleansing process, as it carries wastes from the body through urine and sweat, stimulates peristaltic movement to eliminate the bowels, and hydrates the lymphatic system, which is the body's plumbing.

Create a basic morning and evening routine for simple self-care, with regular times for sleeping and waking. Take ten minutes in the morning and evening for self-care practices. In the morning, take time to clean each of the senses—eyes, ears, nose, and tongue—in addition to eliminating wastes (bowels and bladder). In the evening, take a warm bath, practice deep belly breaths (see page 97), or sit in stillness before bedtime. The simple daily routine below for morning is part of a daily routine of cleansing practices, or *dinacharya*, that is recommended in week 4, and we will add more specific morning and evening self-care recommendations for your type in chapters 8 to 10.

SIMPLE DAILY ROUTINE FOR MORNING

- Drink warm water.
- Eliminate waste from the bowels and bladder.
- Observe the tongue and coating, then swish one teaspoon of sesame oil in the mouth for five to ten minutes and spit it out (see oil pulling, right); brush teeth and scrape the tongue (with a tongue scraper or edge of a spoon).

÷ Splash the eyes with cool water—or if they are red or irritated, spritz with rose water.

÷ Use a neti pot to clear the sinuses of excess mucus or use a few drops of sesame oil in each nostril if you have no congestion.

÷ Place one or two drops of sesame oil in each ear and massage with a fingertip.

oil pulling

Swishing and gargling oil in the mouth is a classic Ayurvedic practice to keep the teeth and gums healthy. Sesame oil is often used because of its anti-bacterial properties, but coconut oil can be substituted if the flavor of sesame is unpalatable. You can also dilute the oil with a small amount of warm water if you do not like the texture in your mouth. This daily maintenance is reported to cleanse the body of some toxins via small capillaries under the tongue in the same way that oil is used to cleanse the skin, our largest organ of elimination, by attracting lipophilic substances that often store toxins in our bodies (see chapter 11 for a description). For more detailed information, refer to Dr. John Douillard's website Lifespa.com.

WEEK 4
— *dietary cleanse for your type* —

The fourth week incorporates a dietary cleanse by eating a vegetarian diet that eliminates heavier food choices like cheese, bread, and pasta. For this week, you will choose one cleanse—grounding, lightening, or cooling—and follow the recommended recipes and lifestyle practices for it (see chapters 8 to 10). Choose the right cleanse for you based on your **current predominant imbalance** (use the Imbalance Checklist from the appendix to determine your imbalance; see page 197.) Choose the grounding cleanse for a Breeze imbalance, the cooling cleanse for a Fire imbalance, and the lightening cleanse for a Mountain imbalance. If you have more than one predominant imbalance, see the Cleansing Table (page 198) to decide which cleanse is right for you. If you have no predominant imbalance, choose a cleanse based on your constitution with mindful consideration of the season (see page 199).

Once you choose your cleanse, read through the appropriate chapter to make sure that it feels right for you, and read through chapter 7 to find tips to make food preparation simple. Each dietary cleansing chapter has recipes specific to one body-mind type or season, but every recipe also has variations for the other body-mind types. For example, you can modify any of the recipes in the lightening cleanse for the Fire type. If you have a predominant Mountain imbalance but know that you cannot handle strong heating spices because of your Fire constitution, use the lightening cleanse with the Fire modifications. This will give you the information you need to adjust your cleanse and make it fitting for you.

FINAL CLEANSING DAYS

The final three days following week 4 incorporate digestive cleansing practices. You will eat **only foods from the**

Basic Cleansing Staples section in chapter 7 and drink **only warm water or warm herbal teas** from the cleanse you chose in week 4. This will give the digestive system a break and strengthen the digestive fire enough to burn up ama and toxins in the digestive tract. Choose only the following:

+ whole and freshly cooked foods
+ warm, simple foods
+ warm or room-temperature drinks

It is also a time to rest and give the body and mind a break from activity. Eliminate all exercise and yoga (except Bed Yoga; see below); choose gentle breathing practices and meditation from the self-care section of chapter 8 (see page 97); take a break from all electronics and mental stimulation, and rest as much as possible. Avoid the following:

+ exercise, vigorous breathing practices, or strenuous activities
+ a busy schedule, including excessive activities or movement
+ mental work or stimulation from computers, cell phones, television, and other electronic devices

Continue all other daily self-care practices for your type, including oil massage or raw silk massage. This is an ideal time to receive Ayurvedic bodywork therapies (see pages 201 to 202) specific to your imbalance if you have access to a practitioner.

The last three days of digestive cleansing involve an Ayurvedic mono diet of foods from the basic staples. If digestion is a challenge for you, to simplify even further, you can limit what you eat to kitchari. The most important part of these three days is eating foods that are easy to digest, so listen to your body and make changes if you are having digestive discomforts. As the body eliminates toxins, you may experience other bodily discomforts, such as aches and pains, headaches, nausea, or excessive heaviness or feeling of exhaustion; these cleansing reactions are natural and will pass. You should feel a lightness in the body by the end of the 31-day protocol.

TRANSITION TIME

After the final cleansing days, it is time to return slowly to your normal routine. Ending your cleansing time by jumping quickly back to many stimulating or dulling foods, heavy foods, or foods inappropriate for your type or the

BED YOGA

During my panchakarma in India, I was advised to take complete rest—no activity or exercise, including yoga. But spending five weeks with little movement was challenging, so we compromised by doing only the stretches we could do gently and comfortably in bed—reclining, supported, and relaxing poses for the most part, with an occasional twist, arm stretch, or a seated forward fold. This turned out to be my favorite yoga for a long time. Try this during your cleanse, but if it is difficult to do in bed, it is probably too much for the final days of digestive cleansing.

modifications of the cleanse

When the basic practices from the 31-day protocol become part of your everyday life, consider modifying the protocol to make the digestive cleansing section longer. Combine all of the practices from the first four weeks into one or two weeks so the digestive cleansing phase is seven to ten days instead of three. Once you have accomplished this without cleansing reactions, listed to the left, you are ready for the deeper cleansing practices in chapter 11 and should consult an Ayurvedic physician or practitioner for guidance.

In the first week following your cleanse, keep it simple—both in diet and in activity. Try not to jump full force into everything. Start with gentle or moderate exercise and yoga, and for Mountain types, move back to vigorous exercise only when you are feeling your usual strength. Try to maintain the daily self-care practices you find helpful and make routines for health and balance a mainstay in your life. Leave out the need for perfection (Fire types, especially) and try to make your daily routine feel supportive and full of ease.

In the second week after the cleanse, reincorporate foods such as meat if you choose to consume it, but remember that it is a concentrated food and keep portions small. You can indulge a little more with richer foods, but notice the effect that these choices have on your body, energy, mind, and emotions. As you cleanse and become more balanced, the foods you once enjoyed may or may not be right for you. Leave some flexibility in your mind for the idea that certain food choices will no longer work for you. This is a sign of progress—that the practices of awareness about food and the cleanse have made a permanent change and you may experience a "new normal."

Finally, use some or all of the awareness practices from the protocol in everyday living. Use the practices of "simple eating" to remind yourself to listen to your own wisdom. Come back periodically to the simple diet plans from week 4 and the basic staples for each season or when your food choices have gone astray—even if you do not have time for the final cleansing days. This happens to all of us when we are busy, stressed, challenged emotionally, or out of our natural routine or environment. Nothing feels better to me after a week of travel than simple, home-cooked meals like kitchari (see pages 79 to 80). I actually crave it!

season could be detrimental to your health. Start by returning for a few days to the dietary cleanse you used in week 4 and choose mostly warm, cooked foods.

Introduce some heavier, more nourishing foods such as mushroom or bone broth (if you eat meat) at the end of the first week. Include raw foods only if appropriate for your type and the season, but be attentive to how your body feels with each new food you add. Notice if digestion feels easy or disturbed, so that you can continue to make food your medicine. Also, pay attention to your tongue coating every day and see if you can use your body's wisdom to help you make mindful food choices.

CHAPTER SEVEN

magic in the kitchen

—

tips for effortless cooking & recipes for basic cleansing staples

tHE RICE COOKER IS THE ULTIMATE in one-pot cooking. Ayurveda explains that foods that are cooked together are more digestible. That means that a grain, a bean, and an assortment of vegetables cooked separately are harder to digest than the same ingredients cooked together in one pot of soup. I found that doing this improved the quality of taste as well as the texture of my dish. Another big benefit of the one-pot cooking: fewer dishes to clean!

If you do not think you have time in your day to prepare all of your own meals, think again. Five minutes in the kitchen is all you need to prepare a pot of kitchari and press the button on the rice cooker. If you take some time once or twice a week to prepare the basic ingredients—like chopped vegetables and spice mixes— then fifteen or twenty minutes is all the time you need in the kitchen. You can prepare 80 percent of the recipes in this cookbook using a rice cooker.

For me, the rice cooker was a revolution in the kitchen. My husband purchased one at a tag sale for thirty-five dollars, and when he brought it home, I had no idea what to do with it. Being adventurous in the kitchen, I knew that I could put it to use. It sat around for a few weeks until I had time to read the manual and figure out what all those buttons could do. Then it took a few more weeks to try out different combinations of food and learn how much water to add and which settings would work for cooking my favorite grains, beans, and veggies. Eventually, I realized

THE MAGIC

Ah, the sound of birdsong in the morning: the first bit of stimulation from the outside world calling me to leave the inner world of nightly dreams. I take a few deep breaths and roll back and forth, stretching from side to side as my body awakens. Gratitude arises for another day, for the warm body of my husband cuddled up beside me in bed, for the sweet baby still asleep down the hall, for sleep itself. Then another busy day with all the activity, planning, "to-do" lists, and multitasking of modern life begins.

I rise and take five minutes of self-care in the bathroom before I head down to the kitchen. It's 6:28 a.m. I fill a kettle with water and place it on the stovetop next to a small pot that I fill with some frozen berries, a banana, and just enough water to cover the fruit. The rice cooker next to me on the counter sings a cheerful line of "Twinkle, Twinkle Little Star" to signal its completion, and that lets me know it's 6:30.

I empty the steaming contents of the cooker into a blender, then rinse out the pot and refill it with lunch ingredients: rice, mung beans, pre-chopped carrots and zucchini, frozen peas, a scoop of spice mix, a scoop of ghee, a squeeze of lemon, and a pinch of salt. I fill the pot with water, place it back in the rice cooker, and set the timer for lunch and again the cooker sings its song.

I turn my attention back to breakfast. I add hot water to the blender and mix the porridge ingredients until smooth and creamy. Mmm, the smell of rice, almonds, dates, and sweet spices makes my tummy growl and my appetite call urgently. Oh, patience, little fire, just one more thing to do. I make a pot of tea and my cooking day is done. It's 6:40 a.m.

Our lunch will be ready at the programmed time, 11:30 am. I can serve it with chutney that I made last Sunday, a little chopped cilantro, and lime. The rest will stay warm in the rice cooker for dinner. I can water-sautee some veggies or bake a sweet potato to complement the rice dish, or for variety, I may puree the veggies with the rice to make a soup. I might spend fifteen minutes in the kitchen again later in the day, for a total of thirty minutes of cooking and three delicious, nutritious, organic, homemade, meals cooked with love for my family. Not too bad!

that this one piece of equipment with its programmable timer and various settings for white rice, brown rice, softer and harder rice, porridge, or quick cooking would allow me to cook 80 percent of my normal staples with 90 percent less work. It was my new best friend!

In the beginning, I would cook the mung beans and rice together in the rice cooker and then water-sautee the veggies separately. I would warm ghee in another pan with spices to lightly roast them and release their aroma, and then combine it all together. That worked great, but I wanted the convenience of the rice cooker to follow me beyond my kitchen. I wanted to be able to take my new best friend on the road when we traveled, so I started combining all the ingredients in one pot to cook together. It turned out wonderfully! We cooked in hotels, yoga studios, and even massage rooms. It went with us everywhere we traveled to teach and work.

I have used several rice cookers over the years and they all reduce your time in the kitchen. Of course, I have found that some features matter more than others. A programmable timer is the function that is most important to me. I can place all of the ingredients for breakfast in the cooker and then set it for the morning—or if I know I will be gone all day, I program it for dinner. With my current cooker, I just set the time that I want it to be done—the simplest option with the least room for error. Other timers have you calculate and program the number of hours until you want the cooking to start. Personally, I don't want to think that much when I am in a hurry.

Another valuable feature is a variety of settings. Rice cookers that have only one setting work, but it is a challenge to get the food to cook thoroughly without drying the top portion or burning the bottom. The cooker I use now has ten settings, from sushi rice to sweet rice. Most people will not use that many settings, but one or two variations are worth the money you will pay for them. Some rice cookers can also double as a slow cooker.

When using any rice cooker to prepare rice, the standard formula is to add one cup of rice and then fill the cooker with water up to the "1" mark inside the pot. It is not necessarily equivalent to the "one cup rice to two cups water" ratio used in stovetop cooking. Because mung beans are harder than rice and require more water to cook, use one cup of kitchari (mung bean and rice mix) and fill to the "2" mark with water (essentially doubling the amount of water to the amount of rice). Each cooker is different and the amount of water for different types of rice is typically marked inside the pot. You will have to experiment with a new rice cooker to determine the correct amounts of rice and water, and to determine what consistency you prefer for your dishes. You can add extra water to make a dish soft like porridge or add less water for firm, differentiated grains or beans.

WEEKLY PREPARATIONS
— and stocking the pantry —

Organization and planning make your time in the kitchen practically effortless and your month of cleansing more enjoyable. Plan one time every month when you can prepare all the basic spice mixes, nectar, spiced honey, and even tea blends. Choose one or two times during the week when you can devote thirty minutes or more to make a shopping list, chop vegetables, mix up sauces or dressings, and make chutneys. With these items prepared, your main dish will take five minutes to assemble using the rice cooker, oven, or stovetop. When using the rice cooker, you can leave the kitchen and come back when it is time to eat. You can use the oven similarly if you have a "stop time" setting. Using the stovetop you will spend fifteen to thirty minutes checking on the food and stirring. That's it. I have learned to make large batches of soup every time I cook so that I can freeze a portion for days when I don't have time to cook.

Cook as many of your own meals as you can throughout the dietary and digestive cleansing protocol—the fourth week and beyond—and, if it is affordable, buy a rice cooker to make it as easy as possible. The investment in your health (and sanity) is worth it. Now the only step left is to make sure that you have all of the ingredients appropriate for your cleanse.

When preparing for your cleanse—or any week—look at the "Eat More" list of ingredients appropriate for your type and stock your cupboards with those items. Keep whole grains and legumes in large glass jars with sealed lids for easy viewing and access. Order the staples you use the most in bulk, including grains, legumes, spices, and teas (see resources for suggested retailers) to limit shopping trips and reduce your costs.

When it comes to fresh produce, see what is in season in your area at a farmers' market or local co-op. Buy more of those foods to easily attune to the seasonal changes.

To keep greens and herbs fresh longer, cut off the tips of the stems and place in a glass of water (as you would with flowers), then cover with a plastic bag and store in the fridge. You do not need to refrigerate root vegetables, but store them in a cool, dark place (especially potatoes) for a longer shelf life. Keep fresh fruit available for snacking and always wash them before consuming.

COOKING TIPS

I have very few secrets in my cooking practices, but my family, friends, and guests always compliment the simple foods I prepare. I have three suggestions from Ayurveda that I rely on to produce excellent results. Give them a try and I think you will be able to taste the difference.

six tastes in each meal

Include all six tastes in each meal to improve satiation and prevent cravings. I take it one step further and include all six tastes in each recipe, even if it is only a pinch of something. In the recipes of this book, the grains are sweet, the beans are astringent, and the vegetables are a mix of bitter, astringent, pungent, or sweet (each has its predominance). The pungent taste usually comes from spices and you add the sour taste with a squeeze of lemon or lime or a splash of vinegar (usually apple cider vinegar because it is less acidic than others). A savory dish will often have a sweet chutney or sweet-and-sour sauce to complement the dish and add any flavor that is missing. I do feel the difference in my level of contentment when I follow this practice.

energizing food

Use your hands to energize the food you are preparing. Each one of the fingers is related to one of the elements— ether, air, fire, water, and earth—so using your hands to hold, mix, or otherwise touch the food will energize it with

leftovers

Ayurvedic texts recommend avoiding leftovers, because of the *tamasic*, or dulling effect, on the body and mind. Yes, it is true that you can taste the difference in freshly cooked foods and those that have been in the refrigerator overnight—some of the food's prana, or energy, is lost. We do, however, have the power of refrigeration, which was not possible when the classic texts were written. I imagine that the leftovers they referred to may have begun to ferment and decompose. I believe it is better to eat your own food, prepared with love and frozen or refrigerated, than any other alternative. I keep to a one-night rule for most leftovers.

those potencies. I use my hands to measure ingredients like grains and beans, and my fingers or palm to measure spices. It is easy to do and results in fewer dishes to wash.

I keep my staple grains in large glass containers that I can reach into with both hands for scooping. We are all different, so at first, use a measuring cup to find out what each measurement looks like in your hand. With my relatively small hands, a one-hand scoop of grains is about ¼ cup, a two-hand scoop is about ½ cup, and a heaping two-hand scoop is 1 cup. Experiment and have fun; touch your food and use your senses. It will nourish you and make the food taste better.

love and gratitude

While you are touching your foods in preparation, remember to put in the love. This is the most important practice in the kitchen—for this reason Ayurveda recommends eating only food that was prepared by someone who loves you. Keeping a calm and quiet environment in the kitchen is important, but so is allowing yourself to experience your senses, enjoy the process, and have fun. If you enjoy the process of cooking, it will nourish you as you prepare and eat the food. If you do not love to cook, then at the very least make sure that you have enough time so that you do not feel rushed or irritable in the kitchen. With any luck, these tips will make preparations so easy that you may grow to love cooking.

BASIC CLEANSING STAPLE RECIPES

From an Ayurvedic perspective, the simpler the diet, the better the cleansing effect. In traditional Ayurvedic cleanses, the following staples are the only foods consumed for several weeks or months. In fact, Ayurvedic practitioners often advise us to eat bland foods during panchakarma to avoid overstimulating the senses. The staples consist of mostly calming foods that are easy to digest and well cooked to give the digestive system a break.

You can use these recipes at any time during your 31-day protocol. They are especially good during the fourth week, when you can incorporate them into any of the cleanses. These staples are the exclusive diet for the final three days of the Ayurvedic mono diet, or digestive cleansing days. As you progress over time with your seasonal cleansing, consider using less variety in the diet and using mostly staples for the duration of the 31 days.

kitchari

Kitchari is a nourishing dish made with equal parts mung beans and basmati rice often recommended as the ideal food in Ayurvedic cleansing and rejuvenation. The mung bean is the smallest, lightest, easiest bean to digest, and combined with basmati rice, it makes a complete protein that is easy to digest. It is mildly spiced to support healthy digestion, so more bodily energy can be devoted to the cleansing process. The ingredients in kitchari are also calming in nature, so the end result is a body and mind that are still, stable, and free of cravings. This combination is not too heating or cooling in nature; it is tri-doshic, or equally balanced.

Basmati rice is a brown or white aromatic whole grain. After harvesting, only the hull is removed, so it retains all of its natural nutrients, bran, and fiber. White basmati rice is milled a second time to remove the bran, reducing its nutritional content but making it easier to digest. The brown version has a heartier, nuttier taste, but since it is slightly harder to digest, it can be used for kitchari only when the digestive fire is strong and balanced.

Mung beans (*Vigna radiata*) have three varieties and many natural colors—green, yellow, olive, black, brown, or purplish-brown. The most common is green, and it is sold whole, or intact; split (appearing green); or split with the skins removed (appearing pale yellow). I have also observed a smaller, shiny, bright-yellow version of split yellow mung beans.

The split yellow mung is so soft that it can easily turn to a smooth soup when cooked. In kitchari, this bean may lose its shape and become homogenously mashed with the rice. This is the best bean for those who have a delicate digestive tract, for deep cleansing, or for rejuvenation when the digestive fire is weak.

Split green mung beans have more fiber due to their skins, and require more water to cook thoroughly. When cooked with rice, they maintain their shape. I have heard that the added fiber is better for Breeze digestion or those with a history of constipation, to add bulk to the stools. To me, it feels slightly rough. If you feel this roughness, either choose the split yellow version or add more ghee and spices.

The whole green mung bean looks like a small, perfectly round green pearl. It is more dense and solid than both split beans, but faster to cook and easier to digest than other legumes like pinto or black beans. It is perfect to use in soups, as the added water content will soften the bean thoroughly.

You can use any of these beans in kitchari—and you can choose the type of grain according to the needs of each person eating it. Changing the amount of water in the recipe varies the consistency from a firm grain to porridge to a soup. This recipe uses white basmati, split yellow mung, and a tri-doshic spice mix. Variations appear for each type, but you can also adjust the recipe to your liking. *continued on page 80 »*

kitchari, continued

YIELD · FOUR 1-CUP (200 G) SERVINGS (UP TO SIX SERVINGS WHEN MADE INTO SOUP)

3–4 cups (705–946 ml) water

½ cup (95 g) white basmati rice

½ cup (92 g) split yellow mung beans

¼ cup (25 g) chopped asparagus

¼ cup (33 g) chopped carrots

¼ cup (25 g) chopped cauliflower

¼ cup (30 g) chopped yellow squash

1 tablespoon ghee (7 g) or coconut oil, if you prefer a vegan option

1 tablespoon (7 g) Simple spice mix (see page 86)

1 teaspoon salt (7 g)

splash of apple cider vinegar or a squeeze of lemon

SERVE WITH:

1 sliced lemon or lime

¼ cup (4 g) chopped cilantro

salt

chutney (see page 85)

One-pot cooking method: Place the water in a large saucepan and bring to a boil on high heat. Use 3 cups (705 ml) of water for a firmer consistency of grain, 3½ cups (825 ml) if you would prefer a porridge-like consistency, and 4 cups (946 ml) if you want a soup-like consistency. Add all of the remaining ingredients and stir. Then reduce the heat to low and simmer for 30–35 minutes covered. Stir occasionally and look for the desired consistency. Serve with sliced lemon, chopped cilantro, salt, and chutney to include all six tastes in one meal.

NOTE: Cooked kitchari congeals as it cools. If it congeals into a dense mass, reconstitute it to a pleasing texture simply by adding water and mashing it when you warm it up.

THE RULE OF INVERSE PROPORTION

The more complicated your physical, emotional, or spiritual life, the simpler your diet should be. This is a simple rule I made up, based on Ayurvedic principles. When we are experiencing physical or emotional stress or are directing our energy to spiritual exercises, our energy is going to manage those stressors or support those exercises, diverting it from our digestive system. Therefore, during these times, it is beneficial to eat a diet that is simple to digest as well as nourishing.

In Ayurveda, we understand that any food can act medicinally or as a poison— poison, in this context, being anything that hinders digestion. And medicine? That's anything that supports it. Kitchari not only provides nourishment for the body, but because of its spice combination, also benefits digestion. This makes kitchari a food of choice for times of stress on the body or the mind. —DR. CLAUDIA WELCH

breakfast porridge and konji

This whole-grain porridge is a staple breakfast for cleansing but is easy to prepare and enjoy in any season. You can modify the recipe for each type or season by choosing the appropriate grain, spice, and oil to deliver the necessary qualities. Konji is a thinner version of the porridge used in times of cleansing or weakness to make the food easier to digest. Konji can also be a healthy meal replacement or snack for busy times when the pace of your life makes it impossible to stop for a full meal.

YIELD · 3 CUPS (660 G) PORRIDGE; 4-6 CUPS (946-1425 ML) KONJI

1 cup (180 g) basmati rice or other grain

3 cups (705 ml) water (depending on the grain)

3 dates, soaked in water overnight and pitted

1 tablespoon (7 g) Sweet Milk spice mix (see page 86)

1 teaspoon ghee (2.3 g)

pinch of salt

squeeze of lemon

FOR KONJI:
additional 1–3 cups (235–705 ml) of water

One-pot cooking method: Combine the rice or grain and 2 cups (475 ml) of water in a large saucepan and cook on medium-high heat until the water boils. Reduce heat to low, stir, and simmer for 15 minutes. Add the remaining ingredients during the last few minutes of cooking, stir, and continue cooking until all the water is absorbed. Transfer to a blender, add the remaining 1 cup (235 ml) of water, and blend first on low, then on high for 1 minute until the porridge is creamy and smooth. Add more water if needed to achieve the desired consistency. The porridge should pour out of the blender when complete.

FOR KONJI: Use an additional 1–3 cups (235–705 ml) water to achieve a drinkable liquid. With more water it will resemble a nut milk or grain milk, but with less water it will be the consistency of a smoothie. In times of weak digestion or illness, use the thinner variety.

CAUTION: Leave the blender lid ajar or remove the round center insert when blending hot items. The heat will create expansion and pressure inside the blender and could cause the lid to pop off while blending.

BREEZE: Use heavier grains like brown basmati rice for porridge when the digestive fire is strong. Drink konji when the digestive fire is weak.

FIRE: Use basmati rice or quinoa for porridge and konji. Konji makes an ideal snack to satisfy hunger between meals.

MOUNTAIN: Use lighter grains like quinoa or millet and have konji for breakfast when lightening the diet.

ghee (clarified butter)

Ayurveda considers ghee, or clarified butter, one of the most important food-medicines. When butter is heated, the thick and sticky milk solids separate from the clear, golden liquid that is ghee. You can strain the ghee out and use it in place of oil for cooking or as a garnish on grains, beans, or vegetables. It lubricates the digestive tract's mucous membranes, helps regulate digestion, lubricates the joints, and increases healthy cholesterol. Ghee is also used in Ayurveda to carry other herbal food-medicines deeper into the body, as ghee has the ability to penetrate into subtle and minute channels.

YIELD · APPROXIMATELY 2 CUPS (450 ML); YOU WILL LOSE A LITTLE GHEE WHEN STRAINING, SO IT IS USUALLY JUST SHORT OF 2 CUPS

1 pound (450 g) unsalted butter

Place the butter in a medium saucepan and warm on medium-low heat for 15–20 minutes. The milk solids will start to foam up on top of the clear liquid when the butter melts, and a bubbling sound will be audible as the water evaporates out of the butter. Around the 15-minute mark, the milk solids will start to sink and brown on the bottom of the pan. At this time, the bubbling sound will stop, signaling that the ghee is almost finished. A second foaming will happen after the ghee becomes quiet, but this foam has thin, clear bubbles opposed to the thick, white, chunky milk solids from the earlier stage. This is the proper time to remove the ghee from the heat. It is of utmost importance to watch the ghee carefully during this time, as it can burn within a minute if left on the heat after the process is complete.

Remove the ghee from the heat and let it cool for 30 minutes. While it is still liquid, strain the ghee through a fine-mesh metal strainer or cheesecloth into a glass jar with a lid. Allow the ghee to cool and solidify completely before covering with the lid. You do not need to refrigerate the ghee as long as you keep moisture out of it. Use a clean, dry spoon each time you take ghee from the jar and then cover it immediately. Moisture in the ghee can allow bacteria to grow, so maintaining cleanliness is important.

chutney

Chutney is a side dish or condiment served with savory dishes. Each of these recipes has all six tastes but is predominantly sweet in flavor to satiate the desire for sweet throughout the day. The fruit's sugar content acts as a preservative, so you can refrigerate a large batch of chutney for a week. The first chutney here is better for the Breeze, the second for the Mountain, and the third for Fire, but a small amount of any chutney is acceptable for all types.

YIELD · 1½ TO 2 CUPS (375-500 G) CHUTNEY

RAISIN COCONUT CHUTNEY

1 cup (145 g) Thompson or flame raisins

½ cup (85 g) coconut

2 soaked and pitted dates

water, enough to cover fruits

1 teaspoon (2.3 g) ghee

1 teaspoon (2 g) fennel seed

pinch of salt

¼ teaspoon ground cardamom

¼ teaspoon ground ginger

squeeze of lemon

⅛ cup (7 g) chopped mint

APPLE CRANBERRY CHUTNEY

1 red or green apple, chopped

½ cup (60 g) dried cranberries

water, enough to cover fruits

1 teaspoon (2.3 g) ghee

1 teaspoon (2.1 g) whole cumin seed

¼ teaspoon ground cinnamon

pinch of salt

squeeze of lemon

⅛ cup (7 g) chopped parsley

1 teaspoon fresh grated ginger

COCONUT CILANTRO CHUTNEY

½ cup (40g) shredded coconut

3 soaked and pitted dates

1 teaspoon (5 ml) coconut oil

1 teaspoon (2.1 g) whole cumin or fennel seed

½ cup (120 ml) coconut milk

½ cup (120 ml) water

pinch of salt

¼ teaspoon Sweet Milk spice (see page 86)

½ cup (8 g) chopped cilantro

For any of these recipes, place all dried and fresh fruits in a small saucepan and add just enough water to cover them. Simmer on medium-low heat uncovered for 15 minutes or until 90 percent of the water is absorbed. While the fruits are cooking, combine the ghee or oil and whole seeds in a small skillet and heat on low until the seeds start to brown and release their aroma (5–10 minutes). Turn off heat and combine the cooked fruits, roasted seeds, and all remaining ingredients in a blender or food processor. Blend on low for 30 seconds to 1 minute to make a chunky sauce. Serve warm in a colder season or cool for 20 minutes before serving in a warmer season. When using refrigerated chutney, take it out 30 minutes before a meal so that it can return to room temperature.

CAUTION: Leave the blender lid ajar or remove the round center insert when blending hot items. The heat will create expansion and pressure inside the blender and could cause the lid to pop off while blending.

spice mixes

Each spice mix is an appropriate blend for your type or your imbalance. You can use a mix with kitchari, individual grains or beans, soups, or vegetable mixes. If cooking for several individuals in your family with different body-mind types, use the Simple spice mix, which is tri-doshic. The first four blends are for use with savory dishes, and the Sweet Milk spice is for porridges, chutneys, or milk drinks.

YIELD · 24 SERVINGS, 1 OUNCE EACH

vata

WARM THE BREEZE:

4 parts turmeric

3 parts coriander

2 parts cumin

2 parts ginger

1 part hing

Pitta

CALM THE FIRE:

4 parts turmeric

3 parts coriander

3 parts cumin

2 parts fennel

Kapha

LIFT THE MOUNTAIN:

4 parts turmeric

3 parts ginger

3 parts mustard seed

2 parts paprika

1 part cumin

1 part coriander

SIMPLE:

3 parts turmeric

3 parts cumin

3 parts coriander

2 parts mustard seed

1 part hing

1 part ground ginger or

⅛ teaspoon freshly grated ginger per 1 tablespoon (7 g) of spice mix (added separately each time you prepare kitchari)

SWEET MILK:

4 parts cardamom

4 parts ginger (2 parts when used for the Fire)

1 part nutmeg

1 part cinnamon in warm weather; 2 parts in cold weather

Choose a spice mix and combine all ingredients together.

Each mix can be made in small or large batches and kept in a sealed container to preserve the potency of the spices. A small batch might use 1 teaspoon (2.4 g) per part, but a large batch might use ⅛ cup (14 g) per part.

spiced honey

Mountain individuals can use raw honey or raw, spiced honey as a sweetener for tea, warm milk, or porridge. Taken on an empty stomach, it is also good for clearing congestion from the lungs and sinuses in any body-mind type. Use spiced honey at the first sign of a cold to dry up excess secretion; for that purpose, take 1 teaspoon (6.5 g) once or twice daily.

YIELD · APPROXIMATELY 17 TEASPOONS (85g)

¼ cup (75 g) raw honey

1 tablespoon (5.5 g) ground ginger

1 teaspoon (2.3 g) ground cinnamon

1 teaspoon (2 g) ground black pepper or long pepper

½ teaspoon (1.2g) ground cardamom

Stir all ingredients thoroughly until all dry powders are coated with honey. Keep in a covered container and use a clean spoon with each use.

NOTE: Honey degenerates with high heat. Ancient Ayurveda taught that it becomes a toxic substance to the body when heated and advised against cooking with honey. When adding it to tea, allow the tea to cool for a few minutes first.

QUALITIES OF GINGER

The qualities of freshly grated ginger root are slightly different when it is dried or ground. The fresh root is sweeter and the dried root hotter. A small amount of fresh ginger is even safe for a Fire type when blended with other cooling spices. If the fresh root is available, use it in place of dried ginger in any recipe from this book. I alternate uses throughout the book because many people will not have access to the fresh variety.

lemon-ginger-honey nectar

This little zinger is always a favorite addition to any meal. The ingredients are all heating in nature, so together they stimulate the appetite and improve digestion. You can take nectar as a shot, 1 teaspoon to 1 ounce, (5–25 ml) before a meal or periodically throughout the day to help clear congestion in the lungs or sinuses.

Honey acts as a natural preservative, so I make a large batch and keep it refrigerated for a week or two. It is best to pour the shot and allow it to return to room temperature before serving. Eating or drinking anything colder than room temperature can weaken digestive fire and expend undue energy, because the body has to warm it up before assimilating it into the system.

You can prepare the nectar in different ratios for different individual needs. The standard recipe is three parts honey, two parts lemon juice, and one part ginger juice, but Mountain types can use equal amounts of honey, ginger juice, and lemon juice.

YIELD · 24 1-OUNCE (25 ML) SERVINGS

1-inch (2.5 cm) wide finger-length of ginger, grated or chopped

½ cup (120 ml) water

1 cup (240 ml) lemon juice

1½ cups (510 g) raw honey

Grate the ginger on a ceramic grater or chop in small pieces. If you have an industrial-grade blender, the size of the ginger chunks are not very important. If you have a standard blender, make the pieces of ginger as small as possible. Add the grated or chopped ginger to the blender with ½ cup of water. Blend on high and allow it to sit for 10 to 15 minutes. Blend again, then strain the ginger juice through a cheesecloth or fine-mesh metal strainer. Place the ginger juice, lemon juice, and raw honey in a jar and shake vigorously until the honey dissolves evenly. This may take several rounds of shaking.

NOTE: Use the remaining ginger pulp to make fresh ginger tea.

NAP FOR YOUR HEALTH

Improve the strength of your digestion by lying on your left side for fifteen to twenty minutes after a meal. This short "digestive nap" can help direct more energy to the body's natural process and increase the potency of the digestive juices in the stomach. Limit the nap to 20 minutes and you will wake up feeling refreshed!

tips for your type

BREEZE: Use the standard recipe nectar and take 1 tablespoon to 1 ounce (15–25 ml) before meals.

FIRE: Use the standard recipe nectar and take 1 teaspoon (5 ml) with breakfast and dinner during cleansing only.

MOUNTAIN: Use equal ratios in the nectar 1:1:1 and take 1 ounce (25 ml) before or after meals.

grounding
cleanse & diet

THE PURPOSE OF THIS DIETARY CLEANSE is to gently lighten by consuming a vegetarian diet of whole grains, legumes, soaked nuts and seeds, fresh vegetables and fruits, good-quality oils and ghee, natural sweeteners, and warming spices. The diet is designed to be warming in nature, with well-cooked foods that are predominantly sweet, sour, and salty tastes. It is good for the Breeze constitution or those with a Breeze imbalance.

Daily practices and self-care include yoga poses, meditation, breath practices, and self-massage to calm the nervous system, relax the mind, ease stress, and create a sense of grounding. Use warming, heavy oils for self-massage to reduce the Breeze imbalance. Time away from the busyness and stresses of life is also advised, so that the nervous system can disengage, rest, and rebalance.

DAILY SELF-CARE PRACTICES

The self-care practices that best suit the Breeze individual are gentle. Remember the delicate flower in the meadow? Too much of anything—movement, touch, pressure, or cold—might damage her sensitive system. When taking on new practices, it is better for the Breeze individual to start gradually with one thing at a time, so that the practices can become a regular part of the daily routine during the 31-day protocol and beyond. Too many changes, too quickly will increase the Breeze imbalance instead of bringing balance.

Incorporate the following practices during the fourth week, along with the simple daily routine from chapter 6. These practices are gentle enough to be continued through the final three days of digestive cleansing for anyone, regardless of the cleanse chosen for week 4. They are also appropriate for everyday maintenance throughout the year for a Breeze type or an individual with a Breeze imbalance. Start with a practice that is interesting to you and commit to it for the entire week. If that feels easy, add another one. Continue in this manner and include as many of these practices as you can each day without increasing stress. Even a few minutes devoted to self-care breaks several times a day will make a difference.

oil self-massage

The skin is the largest organ of the body, and every bit of it is intimately connected with nerve fibers, the extensions of the brain and nervous system. Like little fingers, these nerve fibers reach out to the skin to discover the world and respond to our interactions with it. These fibers carry signals for touch, pressure, pain, heat, and cold back to the brain, and each fiber is insulated with a fatty coating, the myelin sheath, which keeps the impulse contained and the delicate nerve protected. If the insulation—which acts like the plastic coating around an electrical wire—is dry, depleted, or thin, the nervous system can feel exposed and overly sensitive. Warm oil applied to the skin feels like putting a blanket of protection over the whole nervous system. It creates a sense of calm, stillness, stability, and grounding.

Ayurveda recommends a daily oil massage for everyone from the very first day of life to the last. The self-massage, called *Abhyanga*, focuses on long strokes over the long bones of the limbs to increase flow of blood and lymph and circular motions around the joints to release tension. The joints have a greater concentration of nerves, so the rhythmic circles applied with warm oil help to calm the nervous system. In fact, warm oil is one of the fastest ways to calm the whole nervous system.

OILS FOR BALANCE

Oil is a food-medicine for the body. It nourishes the skin and penetrates into the subtle channels to open any blockages in the tissues below. It can relieve aches and pains in the muscles with its penetrating action and improve overall circulation of fluids to aid in cleansing the body naturally. According to Ayurveda, the oil is absorbed through the skin and feeds the body in the same way food and

CONTRAINDICATIONS FOR OIL MASSAGE

The metabolic fire, agni, is also present on the cellular level in the body. It must be strong enough to digest the oil applied to the skin, otherwise it could result in the production of ama. For this reason, Ayurveda recommends avoiding oil application when the tongue has a thick coating, in acute illness, when fever is present, and during menstruation.

THE BENEFITS OF HERBALIZED OILS

In Ayurveda, we learn that one of the special properties of oil is that it takes on the qualities of what is cooked in it. Therefore, if we wish to enhance the medicinal effects of massage oils, it is best to use oils that are prepared with herbs that enhance the balancing or medicinal effects we are looking to promote. For example, for Breeze types, it is typically better to use an oil that includes sweet, heavy, warming, and nourishing herbs; for Fire types, use drying, cooling, bitter, and astringent herbs; and for Mountain types, use oil that is prepared with drying, lightening, warming, and rough herbs. We can see that because both Fire and Mountain are oily, it is especially beneficial to use massage oils that are prepared with Fire and Mountain pacifying herbs, so that the oil itself is more likely to have a balancing effect. —DR. CLAUDIA WELCH

water nourish through the digestive tract. It is important to realize that what you put on your skin is absorbed into the body. The common sense rule follows: If you would not put it in your mouth, do not put it on your skin.

Oil that is cold-pressed, organic, and processed without the use of chemicals is best for massage. The qualities of any oil are part of the nourishment and balance delivered through daily self-massage, so choose oil with this in mind. Herbalized oils are often used in Ayurveda to make a base oil more potent and more specific in its action.

❖ Breeze individuals need oils that are warming, calming, and grounding in nature, like sesame, olive, or almond oil. Herbalized vata oil has herbs to balance the Breeze and reduce vata. Ashwagandha Bala oil is a warming formula used for rejuvenation when high vata has depleted the tissues. Mahanarayan oil is a traditional formula that is appropriate for joint rejuvenation.

❖ Fire individuals need cooling and soothing oils such as coconut, sunflower, or safflower. Herbalized pitta oil has cooling herbs to balance the Fire and reduce pitta imbalances. Fire types commonly use Brahmi oil in a coconut base for cooling and calming the mind.

✢ Mountain individuals require heating and stimulating oils like mustard or sesame. Herbalized kapha oil has herbs to balance the Mountain and reduce kapha accumulations. Mahanarayan oil also has properties that help remove congestion from the lungs and sinuses.

Quantity of oil for a massage varies, based on your constitution and current imbalance. Mountain individuals or those with naturally moist or oily skin can use one to two ounces (25–50 ml) per massage. Breeze individuals or those with dry skin can use up to eight ounces (200 ml). Fire individuals fall somewhere in the middle, so an average amount would be three to four ounces (75–100 ml) per massage.

MASSAGE SETUP AND PROCEDURE

Daily oil massage is the fountain of youth that will keep tissues soft, flexible, and healthy as we age. It is a simple practice, but is often set aside if the task of gathering supplies seems too difficult. Acquiring and organizing a few items and keeping them easily accessible will make self-massage easier.

Make sure you also have a warm space, such as your bathroom, where you can relax undressed and uninterrupted for ten to fifteen minutes while you are oiling. Any time of day or night is appropriate for massage, although morning is ideal for cleansing and evening is ideal for relaxing before bedtime. Make sure to allow adequate time so that you do not feel rushed through the process.

Note: Ayurveda recommends oiling before applying heat like a shower or bath, but I know individuals who have experienced serious problems with their plumbing due to oil. Consider oiling after bathing if you have sensitive plumbing. If you would prefer to leave the oil on your body throughout the day, first take a warm bath, shower, or steam to open the pores and then follow with your oil massage. Remember that some oil may get onto your clothing, so refer to the tips below for proper laundering.

tips for removing oil from cloth

In more than two decades of massage practice, I have used many products to aid in removing oil from towels, sheets, and clothing. I recommend Super Washing Soda by Arm & Hammer. When washing oily towels or sheets, use ¼ to ½ cup (55–115 g) washing soda in addition to your regular detergent and wash in hot water on a pre-soak cycle. To clean spots of oil from clothing, add a small amount of washing soda to your detergent and rub into the stain, then wash out in hot water. Use the dryer's low heat setting to dry our oil towels and sheets, to avoid combustion. You will eventually need to replace the towels when they feel oily or moist even after laundering.

oil massage instructions

1- to 8-ounces (25–200 ml) of oil appropriate for your type (see pages 93–94)

4- to 8-ounce (100–200 ml) plastic squeeze bottle or glass container with a well-sealed lid

small bowl

one or two old towels that can get oily

1. Place oil appropriate for your type in a four- to eight-ounce (100–200 ml) sealable glass container or plastic squeeze bottle. You also may want to have a small bowl available to hold and scoop oil after warming it.

2. Run hot water in your bathroom sink and place the oil bottle in the water for a few minutes. The oil should be comfortably warm when it is ready for application. Pour the proper amount of oil into the bowl to make application easy.

3. Place on old towel over a chair or on the floor to create a comfortable sitting area. Note: The towels will eventually build up oil, so dedicate a few old towels for daily massage and see left for how to launder properly.

4. Place a small amount of oil in your palm and apply it to your body. Start anywhere on your body that feels right and try to cover every bit of skin you can reach. It is more important to focus on the speed and intention of your touch than the mechanics or details of the massage. Move slowly for calming (Breeze and Fire types) or vigorously for stimulating (Mountain types), and focus on giving love to each part of your body. The Ayurvedic word for "oil," *sneha*, is also the word for "love."

5. Apply the oil with long up-and-down strokes on your limbs and circular motions around the joints. Use circular clockwise motions at the continued on page 96 »

oil massage, continued

navel, circular motions on the chest and around breasts, and long up-and-down strokes along the spine (as much as you can reach with your hands behind your back). Massage each finger and toe thoroughly.

6. Pour 1- to 4-ounces (25–100 ml) of oil on the top of your head and spread it around your scalp. Use more oil if you are in need of calming the nervous system or slowing down the mind and less oil if you are feeling heavy, dull, or congested. Lean forward and massage your whole scalp with shampooing movements of your fingers. While bending forward, rest your elbows on your thighs or knees so that your shoulders will not feel tired or strained from the

work of massaging. Massage your face and neck using the whole palm to relax tight muscles with special focus on the front and sides of your neck.

7. Relax in the warm room for a few minutes with the oil on your skin.

8. Pat off excess oil with an old towel and make sure your feet are not slippery. (If you are leaving the oil on for the rest of the day, skip step 9.)

9. Take a warm bath, steam, or shower, being extremely careful not to slip. The warm water opens your pores and allows the oil to penetrate deeper into your tissues. It is not necessary to soap your skin, but you can use a mild soap on your hairy parts. If you want to wash your hair, it is best to apply the shampoo directly to your oiled hair before wetting it. This will allow the oil and shampoo to bond, so that the oil will rinse out easily.

10. Take a few minutes to be still, breathe deeply, and notice the effects of the oil massage on your body and mind. The manner in which you start or end your day will set the tone physically and emotionally for everything that follows. A relaxing massage experience in the morning can help you maintain calm throughout the day; before bedtime, it can bring sound, restful sleep.

BREATHING PRACTICES

The deep belly breath and the three-part breath are the foundational steps to all other breathing practices. These are the natural breaths we use as babies and the pattern of breathing we return to in sleep. It brings calming and grounding by sending a signal to the nervous system that it is safe to relax. But in waking hours, the effects of stress, emotional blockages, and constriction of muscles around the rib cage often make our breathing shallow.

The three-part breath, or long breath, is often easier to accomplish lying down at first, but with practice can be done in any position, at any time. Ideally, it is the breath we use every moment of every day. I recommend starting with part 1 and practicing until that is comfortable, then adding the other two parts. Use this breath for a few minutes in bed before sleeping and after waking, and then take breaks throughout the day to remind your body to stay calm.

Sit or lie down in a comfortable position. Notice your breath. Allow it to become slow and deep.

Part 1: Inhale and invite the breath down into your belly and let the lower abdomen (below the navel) expand in all directions, then exhale fully. Expand the space in and around the hips, genitals, and low back, filling the entire bowl of your pelvis with breath. After several long, slow, deep belly breaths, allow the breath to expand upward, toward the lower rib cage.

Part 2: Expand the belly first and then the lower rib cage with each inhalation. You can place one hand on the belly and one on the lower ribs to draw your attention there. As you exhale, try to allow the rib area to let go first, then the belly. Continue for several breaths.

Part 3: Now let the breath move up the body like a wave: Inhale into the belly first, the lower ribs second, and finally into the upper ribs, just below the collarbone, so that the chest lifts. Now allow the wave of breath to flow out from the upper ribs, then from the lower ribs, followed by the belly. Finally, squeeze the navel to the spine to press out all the air. Continue with this breath for several minutes.

MEDITATION

Meditation is a practice to reconnect with the natural and healthy state of the mind—stable, calm, clear, and pure—to witness the true self within. The first step in learning to meditate is concentration exercises to make the mind one-pointed. Tratakam, or candle-gazing, is a concentration practice that can become a meditation. This is an ideal starting place for those new to meditation and also for people with an active imagination or mind who may get lost in their own thoughts with a closed-eye meditation. Practice for a few minutes at a time.

Sit in a comfortable position. Watch the flame of a burning candle. Let your awareness become pointed on the flame. If any thoughts arise in the mind, notice them, but return your attention to the flame. Keep a relaxed body and breath without giving too much attention to either.

Notice if it is easy to still the mind and remain focused or if the mind's activity keeps taking you away from the flame. Continue to watch both the flame and whatever arises in you from the perspective of a witness, as if you were watching a movie. Remind yourself compassionately to bring your awareness back to the flame again and again. Use this practice regularly to create a calm, still, and single-pointed focus in the mind.

YOGA POSES

Yoga postures for balancing the Breeze are calm, steady, slow, grounding, strengthening, warming, and consistent. They stretch and open the spine, low back, hips, back of the legs, and joints. These include seated positions, forward bending postures, gentle movements of the spine and joints, hip openers, and reclining postures. Gentle backbends while lying down can strengthen the low back and core muscles, as can standing postures that focus on grounding.

Precautions: Forward-bending postures can create excess pressure on herniated or bulging discs in the spine or on the vertebrae when osteoporosis is present. To prevent this, bend forward from the hips, with a straight spine.

Try these three postures individually or together:

joint circles

Rotate each joint in circles slowly (ten times in each direction) to create more range of motion and produce more synovial fluid for ease of movement. You can do this in a reclining, seated, or standing position. Include the ankles, knees, hips, wrists, elbows, shoulder, and neck, but note that the knees and elbows will only bend and straighten. Be careful with the neck: Forward bending is safe, but backward movement may pinch nerves of the spine or compress vertebrae. Circle the neck, but bring the head straight across from one shoulder to the other (not backward).

bound angle, or the butterfly posture

Sit on the floor with your legs crossed. If your low back rounds outward or feels tight, sit on a cushion, folded blanket, or a block, so that you can sit up straight. Place the soles of the feet together and let the knees drop out to the sides. If there is strain in the knees, place a pillow under each one for support.

Take a few deep belly breaths and allow the hips and thighs to relax. If this is comfortable, then "flap your butterfly wings" by raising and lowering the knees simultaneously. Return to stillness, then lean forward with a straight back until you feel a stretch in the low back and hips. Breathe deeply and lengthen the spine as you inhale, then sink down deeper into the stretch as you exhale. Finally, allow your back to round as you curl over the legs, finding the stretch that is just right for you, using your hands on the ground for support. Relax here and continue deep belly breaths, then slowly come out of the stretch.

lunge to forward bend

Start in a kneeling position with your torso upright. If your knees are tender, place a blanket under them for padding. Step your right foot forward and place the sole of your foot on the floor in front of you, taking a lunge position (see page 130). Rock forward and backward in this position, feeling the hips opening.

Bend forward and round over the right leg, letting your hands come to the floor for support. (If your hands do not touch the floor, use two yoga blocks—one on each side of the right leg—for hand supports.) Take a few deep breaths and feel the muscles along the spine stretch. Begin to straighten the right (front) leg gently and then release the stretch by bending the knee. Allow your whole body to rock with these alternating movements. Finally, straighten the leg and relax into the stretch along the entire back of the body, including the calf, hamstring, low back, and spine. Breathe deeply and hold for one minute, then slowly release. Repeat this sequence with the other leg.

TIPS FOR SUCCESSFUL DIETARY CLEANSING

These recommendations are geared toward an individual with a Breeze constitution or a Breeze imbalance, to improve health and balance on a daily basis. They are also particularly important during the week of dietary cleansing and the final three days of digestive cleansing. After you have completed the first three weeks of the 31-day protocol and move into the fourth week, follow these suggestions as much as possible.

Meals: Drink a warming tea thirty minutes before each meal and take lemon-ginger-honey nectar (see page 88) immediately before each meal to improve appetite and digestive fire. Take a nap afterward to support the process of digestion (see page 88).

Snacks: If you are hungry between meals, choose cooked fruit with warming spices, warm milk drinks, or warm konji and make sure to allow proper time (thirty minutes for fruit alone; two hours for konji) to digest the snack before your next meal.

Water: Drink only warm water this week. Start your day with a large glass of warm water with lemon, and take self-care breaks to drink water periodically throughout the day—one hour before or two hours after a meal. Reduce water intake in the evening hours, so that it does not interfere with sound sleep.

Rest: Try to be in bed by 9:30 p.m., so that you can be asleep by 10. Make a goal of eight full hours of sleep each night, and try to rise between 6 and 7 a.m.. If your sleep is disturbed during the night, use calming practices from the self-care section to create enough grounding to return to sleep (see pages 91 to 99).

Self-care: Prioritize an evening self-care routine so that heaviness can accumulate in the body and prepare it for sleep. Oil the body at night and then take a warm bath if you have any challenges staying asleep. Oil both morning and night if you have the time and your tongue is free of excess coating. Incorporate as many practices as you can in the morning and at night without feeling rushed. If necessary, stay warm with extra layers of clothing.

Stress-reduction: If you can, take time away from work during this week; the more that you can relax the nervous system, the better your results from the cleanse will be. If not, take self-care breaks periodically during the day to practice deep breaths, yoga poses, or meditation; even five minutes will help. Prioritize the deep breathing exercises as the most important practice every day.

"EAT MORE" LIST
— for the breeze's daily diet and the grounding cleanse —

Choose foods that are **warm, moist, heavy, and oily** in quality and tastes that are **sweet, sour, and salty**.

Eat more of the following:

fruits that are sweet, sour, heavy, or juicy in nature, such as avocadoes, bananas, berries, cherries, figs, grapefruit,

daily schedule

6-7 a.m.	Wake, ideally after eight hours of sleep.
	Do deep belly breaths.
	Drink warm water.
	Eliminate waste from bowels and bladder.
	Do yoga poses.
	Clean the senses; observe the tongue.
	Oil and shower (now or at night; both if time allows).
7:30 a.m.	Drink tea.
8 a.m.	Breakfast.
11 a.m.	Self-care break with deep breaths or yoga poses, followed by water intake.
Noon	Drink tea.
12:30 p.m.	Lunch (your biggest and heaviest meal), followed by a digestive nap (see page 88).
4 p.m.	Self-care break with deep breaths or yoga poses, followed by water intake.
5:30 p.m.	Drink tea.
6 p.m.	Dinner.
8:30 p.m.	Do yoga poses or oil and take a warm bath; do candle-gazing meditation, and put drops of oil in ears.
9:30 p.m.	Consume warm milk drink and prepare for bedtime; go to sleep by 10 p.m.

grapes, lemons, mangoes, sweet melons, oranges, lemons, limes, papayas, peaches, pineapples, and plums. Most fruits are good for the Breeze individual. Cooked fruits are better in a cold season or when the digestive fire is weak.

vegetables that are sweet or heavy in nature, such as asparagus, beets, carrots, cucumbers, garlic, green beans, okra, cooked onions, parsnips, peas, sweet potatoes, yellow squash, zucchini, and yams. *Eat in moderation*: lettuce, leafy greens, sprouts, and spinach. *Eat well cooked*, with oil and proper spices: broccoli, Brussels sprouts, cabbage, cauliflower, celery, kale, potatoes, tomatoes, and winter squashes.

grains that are heavy or warming, such as basmati rice, brown rice, wild rice, oats, quinoa, and wheat

legumes that are easy to digest, such as mung beans, soy, and yellow or red lentils

nuts and seeds if they are soaked, made into nut milks, or cooked, especially almonds and sesame seeds

ghee or raw cow's milk as food-medicines for lubrication and nourishment, if you eat dairy

oils of sesame, olive, and almond

sweeteners that are natural and unprocessed, such as raw sugar, molasses, rice syrup, and, in moderation, honey and maple syrup

condiments that are warming, sweet, sour, or salty, such as basil, lemon, lime, salt, seaweed, and vinegar, and, occasionally, cilantro or mint

spices that are sweet, warming, and calming in nature such as cardamom, curry leaves, ginger, fenugreek, and hing. Use coriander, cumin, fennel, saffron, or turmeric in combination with other warming spices and use cinnamon and nutmeg in moderation.

For non-cleansing times, use mushroom broths or bone broths, (if you consume animal products) to build strength—or beef, chicken, or turkey.

Limit or avoid the following types of foods:

✤ cold, dry, or light in nature

✤ astringent, bitter, and pungent in taste

✤ rough and dry such as crackers, chips, or popcorn

✤ raw, cold, rough, and difficult-to-digest foods, including raw fruits, vegetables, and nuts (except in a warm season or when you are making them into juice or milk)

grounding recipes

The recipes that follow include foods that are warm, well cooked, moist, and oily, to counter the cold, dry, and light qualities of Breeze and create a lighter workload for a delicate digestive fire. The ingredients are mostly calming in nature, with a few stimulating spices and vegetables like onions and garlic used to create more warmth. The spice blends kindle the digestive fire, the heavier root vegetables create a warm and grounded feeling, and whole grains and legumes provide a complete protein that is easy to digest. These recipes are best for the autumn as part of a seasonal diet, throughout the year for those with a Breeze constitution or imbalance, or as part of the grounding dietary cleanse.

indian chocolate spice

Enjoy all the creamy deliciousness of the richest hot chocolate—without the guilt. Since there is no chocolate in this recipe, the magic ingredient here is the powdered root ananta mula, nicknamed "Indian Chocolate" for its rich, earthy, sarsaparilla-spiced flavor. The root's heavy, grounding qualities nourish deeply while satiating the desire for sweet. Combined with warming spices, this drink is perfect as an evening ritual before bedtime or a hand-and-heart-warming answer to the cold of fall.

YIELD · 2 SERVINGS, ½ CUP (120 ML) EACH

1 cup (235 ml) raw cow's milk, fresh almond milk, or hazelnut milk

1 tablespoon (7 g) ananta-mula powder

¼ teaspoon (1.8 g) ginger powder

¼ teaspoon (2 g) cardamom powder

¼ teaspoon (2.3 g) cinnamon powder

⅛ teaspoon (2.2 g) nutmeg powder

1 star anise, whole

1 teaspoon (5 g) ghee

maple syrup to taste

Combine the milk, ananta-mula powder, and spices in a small saucepan and warm on medium heat for 5 to 7 minutes until it starts to gently boil and foam. Remove from the heat, scoop out the star anise, add the ghee, and mix in a blender first on low, then on medium-high. Pour ½-cup to 1-cup (120–235 ml) servings into mugs. Add maple syrup if more sweet taste is desired.

CAUTION: Make sure the blender lid is secure, because the heat will cause expansion and pressure inside the blender and could pop the lid off.

tips for your type

FIRE: Cut spice amounts in half.

MOUNTAIN: Use almond or hazelnut milk, add a pinch of black pepper, and omit sweetener and ghee. Drink in moderation.

so-good-you-can't-stop fresh almond milk

If you have never tasted fresh almond milk, now is the time. It might be hard to imagine the difference between packaged and fresh, but it is comparable to the difference between fast-food and a home-cooked feast. Fresh almond milk is best within three days of preparation. I never need to worry about that, because once I take a drink it is hard to stop. In my house, fresh almond milk is lucky to last one day.

YIELD · 2 TO 3 CUPS (475–710 ML)

1½ cups (210 g) almonds

4–5 dates

1 quart (946 ml) water

¼ teaspoon (0.5 g) Sweet Milk spice (see page 86)

pinch of salt

⅛ teaspoon vanilla extract

maple syrup to taste

In a large bowl, pour water over almonds until they are covered by 1 inch (2.5 cm). Place the dates in a separate bowl and cover in the same manner, then soak both overnight. Drain the almonds and peel the skins off; if adequately soaked, the skin should pop off when squeezed. If not, boil 2 cups (480 ml) of water and soak the almonds again for 1-2 minutes. Place the peeled almonds in the blender and discard the skins.

Strain the dates, but keep the soaking water and remove the pits before adding to the blender. Measure the date water and add enough filtered, spring, or well water to equal 1 quart (946 ml). The purity of the water determines the quality and taste of your milk, so use the best water available. If you have only chlorinated tap water, place 1 quart (946 ml) of water in an open pitcher overnight to evaporate the chlorine.

Place all other ingredients in the blender and puree on the highest setting for several minutes until uniformly blended. To strain, pour the milk slowly through a nut-milk bag or several layers of cheesecloth and squeeze gently to push the liquid through the cloth. I strain the milk twice; first through a fine metal mesh strainer, then through the cloth. Store the milk in a sealed glass container and refrigerate.

NOTE: This whole process takes about 30 minutes, so allow adequate time in your schedule. Remember: the energy used to prepare your food is also part of its nourishment.

tips for your type

FIRE: Drink fresh or use in Turmeric "Latte" (see page 168).

MOUNTAIN: Drink warm in small amounts with extra cinnamon and ginger.

sweet breeze digestive tea

This sweet and simple tea is a great way to stimulate the appetite before a meal or improve digestion with certain foods. Cardamom is a sweet, exotic spice that is calming in nature and improves digestion of hot and cold foods or drinks. Added to coffee, cardamom can counter some negative effects (see sidebar on page 168). It may also improve digestion of cold foods such as ice cream, which can put out the delicate digestive fire of a Breeze due to the heavy and cold qualities. Drink a cup before meals or with sweet treats.

YIELD · 1 QUART (946 ML)

1 teaspoon (2.7 g) fresh grated ginger root

1 teaspoon (3.5 g) dried licorice root

8 whole green cardamom pods

1 quart (946 ml) hot water

Boil water and place all ingredients in a tea ball or metal mesh strainer. Pour the water over the herbs into a thermos. Steep for 10 minutes and serve.

tips for your type

FIRE: Replace ginger with fennel seed.

MOUNTAIN: Do not use licorice.
Sweeten with spiced honey instead.

black rice and cashew porridge

Chewy, creamy, and delicious! My husband tasted a porridge made with forbidden black rice at one of our favorite breakfast places, Haven, in Lenox, Massachusetts. He raved about it for so long that I finally had to try making it. The black rice was perfect—a firm texture that turns chewy, yet creamy when cooked and blended. It is definitely my favorite version of breakfast porridge.

YIELD · THREE TO FOUR ¾- OR 1-CUP (165–220 G) SERVINGS; 3½ CUPS (770 G) TOTAL

3 cups (706 ml) water

pinch of salt

1 cup (190 g) black rice, uncooked

¼ cup (50 g) cashews, soaked

¼ teaspoon (0.6 g) ground cardamom

1 cup (235 ml) oat or almond milk

1 teaspoon (5 g) ghee

4 dates, soaked overnight in water and pitted

FOR GARNISH:
fresh sliced strawberries or mango with mint or cooked apples and pears (see page 170)

Place 2½ cups (580 ml) water and salt in a medium saucepan and bring to a boil on high heat. Add the rice, reduce heat to low, and simmer, covered, for 20 minutes or until all of the water is absorbed. Transfer the rice into a blender and add all other ingredients, plus an additional ½ cup (120 ml) hot water. Blend on low, then high, until porridge is creamy and well blended. To serve, pour into bowls and garnish with your choice of fresh sliced fruit or cooked fruit.

CAUTION: Leave the blender lid ajar or remove the round center insert when blending hot items. The heat will create expansion and pressure inside the blender and could cause the lid to pop off while blending. You can also blend smaller portions to ensure your safety.

NOTE: If your digestion is weak, eliminate the fresh-fruit garnish and eat raw fruit only when it is ripe and in season.

tips for your type

FIRE: Choose cooked apples and pears as a garnish.

MOUNTAIN: Use additional water instead of milk; do not use ghee or dates (use spiced honey for additional sweetness); choose cooked apples and pears as a garnish; and enjoy only occasionally.

gingery oatmeal squares with banana-berry delight sauce

I originally tried a breakfast oatmeal bar at Café Azafran in Delaware. I decided to make a lighter version without eggs, sugar, or heavy dairy products. I incorporated tips I have used in the past when cooking for vegan friends, using bananas and dates as the glue that holds it all together. The flaxseeds also add a slippery quality that helps lubricate the digestive tract and ease the movement of the bowels. It's a perfect warm, nourishing breakfast for the Breeze or during the fall.

YIELD · EIGHT 2-INCH (5 CM) SQUARES

DRY INGREDIENTS

2 cups (160 g) rolled oats, uncooked

⅓ cup (56 g) flaxseeds

⅓ cup (37 g) almond meal

⅓ cup (40 g) oat flour

½ teaspoon (1.2 g) ground cinnamon

1 teaspoon (1.8 g) ground ginger

pinch of salt

WET INGREDIENTS

2 tablespoons (28 g) ghee, melted

1 tablespoon (21 g) maple syrup

1 teaspoon (5 ml) vanilla extract

2 ripe bananas

4 soaked and pitted dates

½ cup (120 ml) oat milk

FOR SAUCE:

1 ripe banana, sliced

2 cups (145 g) sweet berries, any variety

¼ cup (120 ml) water

Combine all dry ingredients in a large bowl or food processor and mix. Add wet ingredients and mix again. If hand-mixing, you may want to puree the bananas, dates, and oat milk in a blender first. Use coconut oil or ghee to grease an 8-inch by 8-inch (20-cm by 20-cm) pan, then spread the oat mixture into the pan and bake on 350°F (Gas Mark 4) for 25–30 minutes. The top of the bars should appear browned and a little crusty when done. Let cool for 10 minutes and cut into squares.

FOR SAUCE: Place all ingredients in a small saucepan and cook on medium heat for 15 minutes, stirring occasionally. The sauce will continue to thicken as more water evaporates, so cook less if you want a juicy sauce or more for a thicker sauce.

TO SERVE: Place one or two oat squares in a bowl and pour oat milk on it and warm banana-berry sauce over the top.

NOTE: The oat squares also make a great snack with Apricot Cherry Sauce (see page 139).

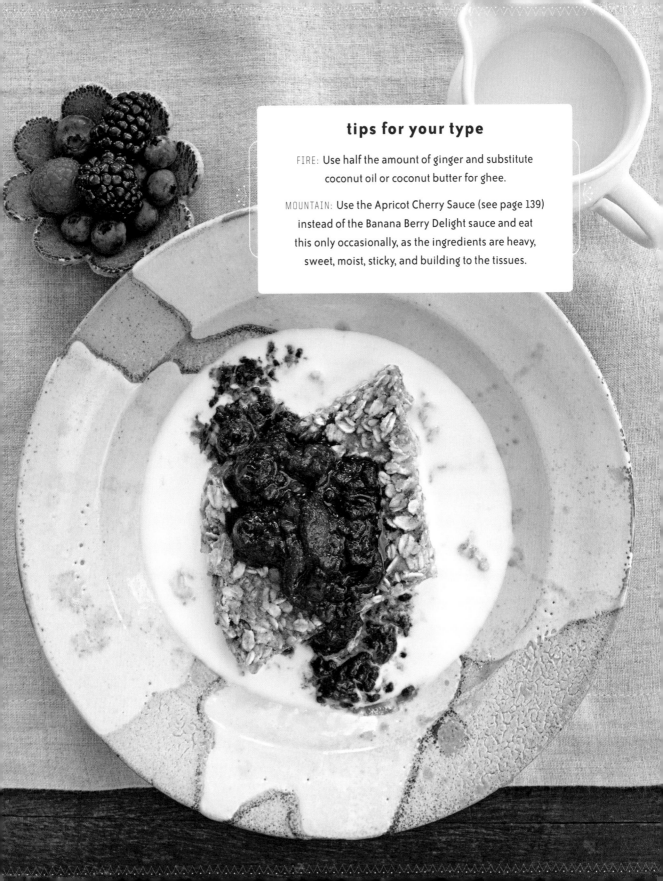

tips for your type

FIRE: Use half the amount of ginger and substitute coconut oil or coconut butter for ghee.

MOUNTAIN: Use the Apricot Cherry Sauce (see page 139) instead of the Banana Berry Delight sauce and eat this only occasionally, as the ingredients are heavy, sweet, moist, sticky, and building to the tissues.

dinner or dessert sweet potato soup

This soup is so sweet and delicious that it can pass as dessert even though it is a satisfying meal. If I am in the mood for a little less sweet, I sometimes use a small butternut squash in place of the sweet potatoes. The simplicity of this soup will win you over if the taste doesn't get you first.

YIELD · FOUR 1-CUP (250 G) SERVINGS

3 medium sweet potatoes or yams, chopped

6 medium carrots, chopped

1 shallot or ¼ of a small onion, chopped

3½ cups (830 ml) water

1 teaspoon (5 g) ghee

pinch of salt

1 teaspoon (2.5 g) ground cumin

½ teaspoon (1.2 g) ground cinnamon

¼ teaspoon (0.5 g) ground nutmeg

½ inch (13 mm) ginger root, grated

FOR GARNISH:
fennel leaf or dill, chopped

Place all ingredients in a medium stockpot and cook on medium heat, covered, for 30 minutes. Transfer to a blender and puree, first on low, then on high, until it is thoroughly creamy. Pour in bowls and garnish with chopped fennel or dill.

CAUTION: Leave the blender lid ajar or remove the round center insert when blending hot items. The heat will create expansion and pressure inside the blender and could cause the lid to pop off while blending. You can also blend smaller portions to ensure your safety.

tips for your type

FIRE: Enjoy in small portions instead of a full meal, because most of the ingredients are warming.

MOUNTAIN: Enjoy in small portions instead of a full meal, because it is heavy and sweet.

the guru kitchari

In Sanskrit the term *guru* means heavy. This version of kitchari is heavy and nourishing, so soaking the grains and beans overnight and using a one-pot cooking method will make these foods more digestible.

YIELD · SIX 1-CUP (220 G) SERVINGS

1 cup (190 g) brown basmati rice

1 cup (184 g) split green mung beans

½ cup (65 g) chopped carrots

½ cup (60 g) chopped zucchini

½ cup (65 g) peas

1 tablespoon (7 g) Warm the Breeze spice mix (see page 86)

1 teaspoon (7 g) salt

1 teaspoon (5 ml) apple cider vinegar or squeeze of lemon

1 tablespoon (14 g) ghee

1 quart (946 ml) water

Rinse the rice and bean mixture a few times and pour off water to remove dirt or sediment. Then add water and let it soak overnight. Combine all ingredients in a medium-size stockpot (3 liter or larger) and cook 45 minutes or until the water is absorbed. You can add more water if you like the kitchari soupy.

tips for your type

FIRE: Use Calm the Fire spice mix instead of the Warm the Breeze spice mix (see both on page 86).

MOUNTAIN: Use occasionally for rejuvenation, but substitute millet or amaranth for the brown rice and use Lift the Mountain spice mix (see page 86).

add it! Use a mushroom or bone broth while cooking this kitchari for non-cleansing times and rejuvenation or when you want to build strength and bulk.

tips for your type

FIRE: Eat in moderation, as the beets can be heating.

MOUNTAIN: Add 2 extra cups (480 ml)
of water to make the soup thinner;
add black pepper; and omit ghee.

golden glow soup

Golden beets are a special treat: a burst of yellow sunshine with a milder flavor than their deep-red cousins. The glow of the beets is enhanced by turmeric, a golden root resembling ginger but with a dark-orange internal flesh, that is commonly dried, ground, and used as a spice in Indian cuisine. For centuries Indian women have used turmeric as their beauty secret for youthful, glowing skin.

YIELD · SIX 1-CUP (250 G) SERVINGS

½ **leek, chopped**

1 tablespoon (14 g) ghee

2 medium golden beets, peeled and chopped

6 medium potatoes, chopped

1-inch (2.5 cm) piece turmeric root, grated, or 1 tablespoon (6.8 g) ground turmeric

1 teaspoon (2.5 g) ground cumin

1 teaspoon (6 g) salt

1 quart (946 ml) water

FOR GARNISH:

1 tablespoon (1 g) chopped cilantro

Add the leek and ghee to a large soup pot and sauté on medium-low for 5 minutes. Add the remaining ingredients and cook on medium-high for 20 minutes or until the vegetables are soft. Pour into blender and puree. Transfer into bowls and garnish with chopped cilantro.

CAUTION: Leave the blender lid ajar or remove the round center insert when blending hot items. The heat will create expansion and pressure inside the blender and could cause the lid to pop off while blending. You can also blend smaller portions to ensure your safety.

add it! For a beautiful splash of color and flavor when you are not cleansing, add a garnish of red beet juice or red beet puree mixed with goat cheese.

1 small red beet, juiced · ¼ cup (35 g) goat cheese

FOR GARNISH: Wash, peel, and juice one red beet, then mix with goat cheese. Pour over individual servings of soup and sprinkle cilantro on top.

Alternately, if you do not have a juicer, chop one-half of a red beet and place in a small saucepan with just enough water to cover it. Cook for 15–20 minutes or until the beets are soft, then pour into a blender with the goat cheese and puree.

what do i have in the kitchen?
water-sautéed veggies

Adding water to a sauté is a technique to combine the moist and soft qualities of steaming with the oily qualities of sautéing. This is ideal for the Breeze who needs moist, soft, oily foods that are well cooked. This technique can also help reduce the amount of oil used to cook foods. A small amount of water adds a slippery quality that can take the place of additional oil, so this can help the Fire and Mountain types when they are limiting oil to lighten or cleanse the body. Use any combination of vegetables you find in the kitchen.

YIELD · FOUR 1-CUP (135 G) SERVINGS

10 Brussels sprouts, halved

4 small orange carrots, peeled and chopped into 1-inch (3 cm) coins

4 small purple carrots, peeled and chopped into 1-inch (2.5 cm) coins

1 teaspoon (5 g) ghee or oil

2 tablespoons (28 ml) water

pinch of salt

¼ teaspoon ground ginger or ¼-inch piece fresh ginger, grated

¼ teaspoon ground coriander

squeeze of lemon or splash of vinegar

Combine chopped vegetables, ghee or oil, and water in a medium sauté pan and cook on medium heat until the water starts to steam. Cover with a lid, reduce heat to low, and cook for 10–15 minutes until all of the water is absorbed and the vegetables are tender to your liking. Add the salt, spices, and lemon or vinegar in the last few minutes of cooking and stir the vegetables to coat evenly. Remove from heat and serve.

TIPS: If you are chopping vegetables for the sauté that are different densities, like Brussels sprouts and green beans, start with the hardest ones first. Start heating the oil and water when you begin chopping and add the vegetables as you chop them. This way the Brussels sprouts get more time cooking and the green beans get less.

tips for your type

FIRE: Use cooling ingredients such as kale and coconut oil.

MOUNTAIN: Use lighter vegetables that are bitter and pungent in taste, such as chard and radishes; add more heating spices like black pepper and paprika; use less ghee or use mustard oil as a substitute; and do not cover with a lid, so that the vegetables retain less moisture.

tips for your type

FIRE: To reduce the amount of heat in this dish, replace beets with celery root, cut the curry leaves in half, and do not use hing.

MOUNTAIN: Use double the amount of spices, use sesame oil instead of olive oil, only a splash of water, and eat as a main dish without any grains.

belly-warming curried roots with tamarind sauce

This is a great fall warmer, when soft comfort foods are appealing. I like to chop the vegetables into large pieces when I make this as a main dish with lemon rice or another grain, but I chop them into tiny pieces when I plan on mixing them with kitchari. Fenugreek, hing, and turmeric make for a powerful digestive aid that can remove excess vata, dispel gas, and remove toxins from the gastrointestinal tract. You can also use this spice mix when cooking beans, to reduce gas and bloating that are common with poor digestion. My belly always feels warm and happy after a meal with curried roots!

YIELD · FOUR 1½ -CUP (270 G) SERVINGS

¼ cup (60 ml) water

2 tablespoons (28 ml) olive oil

6 fresh curry leaves, diced

¼ teaspoon ground fenugreek

¼ teaspoon ground turmeric

¼ teaspoon asafoetida (hing)

1 cup (110 g) chopped parsnips

1 cup (150 g) chopped yams

6 pearl onions or shallots, peeled and chopped

1 cup (225 g) chopped beets, any varieties

½ cup (50 g) chopped fennel root

1 cup (130 g) chopped tricolor carrots

FOR GARNISH:
fresh basil leaves

FOR SAUCE:
4 tablespoons wet tamarind paste

1 cup (235 ml) hot water

1 teaspoon (2.6 g) ground fennel

1 teaspoon (1.8 g) ground ginger

1 teaspoon (2.5 g) ground cumin

⅛ teaspoon ground paprika

⅛ teaspoon chili powder

¼ teaspoon (1.5 g) salt

2 tablespoons (42 g) maple syrup

squeeze of lemon

Mix water, oil, curry leaves, and spices in the bottom of a glass baking dish or covered clay baking pot. Add all chopped vegetables and coat thoroughly in the oil and spice mixture. Bake at 400°F (204°C) for 30–40 minutes, stirring occasionally to recoat the vegetables. In an uncovered baking dish, the vegetables will have a dry and roasted appearance when done and will be fork-tender—better for the Mountain types. When baked in a covered dish, the vegetables will be steamed with a softer and slightly mushy texture, which is better for the Breeze. Baking time will vary; 30 minutes is adequate for finely chopped vegetables, while larger chunks will require 40 minutes or longer. Garnish with fresh basil leaves.

FOR SAUCE: Pour hot water over wet tamarind paste and soak for a few minutes. Stir and press the paste with a spoon or hand to separate the fruit from the seeds and hair-like particles. Combine all other ingredients in a small bowl and strain the tamarind through a fine mesh strainer into the bowl. Press the pulp into and through the strainer and mix the ingredients thoroughly. Pour over individual servings to taste.

beans and greens with cashew miso tofu

Tofu is an easy way to add a little excitement to a simple meal of staples. I think many people avoid tofu because they do not know how to prepare it. It will take on the flavor of any sauce, so the only trick to delicious tofu is to create an interesting marinade. Even before I studied Ayurveda, I noticed that I was relying on three tastes when creating a marinade: sweet, sour, and salty. Now I add a hint of pungent to aid digestion.

YIELD · FOUR 1½-CUP (270 G) SERVINGS

1 cup (192 g) lentils
or adzuki beans, soaked
in water

3 cups (706 ml) water

½ cup (72 g) corn

10 pearl onions

½ cup (70 g) finely
chopped carrots

1 teaspoon (2.7 g)
grated ginger

1 teaspoon (5 g) ghee

½ teaspoon (3.5 g) salt

FOR WATER-SAUTÉ:

1 cup (100 g)
chopped bok choy

1 cup (100 g)
chopped green beans

½ cup (150 g) green peas

2 teaspoons (10 ml) water

¼ teaspoon (1.3 ml)
olive oil

FOR TOFU:

15 ounces (425 g) tofu,
drained and pressed

1 tablespoon (15 g)
cashew butter or tahini

1 teaspoon (5.3 g) miso

1 orange, squeezed

1 tablespoon (15 ml)
liquid aminos

2 tablespoons (30 ml)
olive oil

pinch of paprika and
black pepper

Soak the lentils or adzuki beans in water overnight, drain, and place in a medium stockpot with three cups water. Cook on high heat until the water boils, then reduce heat to low, cover, and simmer for 30 minutes. Add all remaining ingredients, stir, and cook for another 20–25 minutes or until the beans and vegetables are soft and tender. While the beans are cooking, water-sauté the vegetables in a medium skillet with a lid (see page 114).

FOR THE TOFU: Drain the water from the tofu, then slice into three ½-inch (1.3 cm) rectangular slabs. Place one clean towel *continued on page 122 »*

tips for your type

FIRE: Omit onions, black pepper, or ginger
if they cause discomfort.

MOUNTAIN: In the marinade, use tahini instead of cashew
butter, lemon instead of orange, sesame oil instead of
olive oil, and an extra ¼ teaspoon each of paprika, ginger,
and black pepper. Bake the tofu for an extra 5 minutes to
reduce the moisture and heaviness.

beans and greens, *continued*

under the tofu on a cutting board or hard surface and another towel over the tofu. Use a large cookbook to press down firmly and evenly on the tofu for 1 minute, then allow it to stay pressed with the weight of the cookbook for another 10 minutes. To create the marinade, mix the remaining ingredients in a small bowl or on a plate with a rim. Slice the tofu into 1-inch (2.5 cm) strips, soak in the marinade for 5 minutes, then bake in the oven for 20 minutes at 375°F (190°C).

TO SERVE: Ladle ½- to 1-cup (about 90–180 g) servings of beans into a bowl, cover with ½-cup (about 70 g) serving of greens, and top with 4 or 5 strips of baked tofu.

COOKED ONIONS VS. RAW ONIONS

Onions are hot, sharp, and tend to aggravate or increase the Fire imbalance. However, cooking onions brings out their natural sweetness, rendering them easier for the Fire type to tolerate. Cooked onions are okay for the Fire type in moderation, but I have encountered more than one Fire individual who could not tolerate even these. So listen to your own body, and if you feel any burning or digestive discomfort after ingesting onions, leave them out next time.

immune-boosting white bean soup

Herbs de Provence is a blend of garden herbs commonly grown in a region of France and is sold premixed, but you can make your own from fresh herbs. Look for rosemary, thyme, tarragon, basil, oregano, savory, fennel, lavender, marjoram, dill, and chervil at your local farmers' market or grow them in your own garden. The herbs have a strong medicinal quality as well as a strong flavor, so a little bit goes a long way. Enjoy frequently in the fall and winter to boost your immunity.

YIELD · SIX 1-CUP (235 ML) SERVINGS

2 cups (430 g) white beans, dried

1 quart (946 ml) water

¼ cup (60 ml) oat or rice milk

½ cup (75 g) chopped sweet potato

1 cup (71 g) chopped broccoli

1 cup (120 g) chopped zucchini

½ small yellow onion, chopped

½ lemon squeezed

1 teaspoon (0.8 g) Herbs de Provence

1 tablespoon (14 g) ghee

1 teaspoon (7 g) salt

Place beans and water in a stockpot overnight, then discard the water in the morning. Refill water and bring to a boil on high, then reduce heat to medium-low and simmer for 45–50 minutes covered. The beans will absorb 90 percent of the water, so that just a small amount will remain in the bottom of the pan. Transfer half of the beans and all of the liquid from the pot into a blender and puree first on low, then on medium. Add ¼ cup (60 ml) of milk to the blender, so that the soup pours easily. Pour back into the stockpot, add remaining ingredients, and cook on medium-low for 35–40 minutes or until all of the vegetables are softened. Serve with fresh basil or other herbs.

CAUTION: Leave the blender lid ajar or remove the round center insert when blending hot items. The heat will create expansion and pressure inside the blender and could cause the lid to pop off while blending. You can also blend smaller portions to ensure your safety.

tips for your type

FIRE: Omit onion if it creates discomfort.

MOUNTAIN: Leave out the sweet potatoes and ghee, use additional water instead of milk, and add a pinch of black pepper and 1 additional teaspoon of Herbs de Provence.

sweetness of fall

I love the fall harvest and savoring the last burst of brilliance from the sunset-colored root vegetables, buttery squashes, and rich green vegetables. I believe that the same awe-inspiring beauty that accompanies the fall foliage in the Berkshires where I live is packed into the final seasonal abundance. Chopping the vegetables becomes like a meditation that nourishes the eyes before it nourishes the rest of the body.

YIELD · 6 SERVINGS, 1 CUP EACH

1 cup (130 g) chopped carrots

1 cup (130 g) chopped acorn squash

1 cup (130 g) chopped butternut squash

10 Brussels sprouts, cut in half

1 tablespoon (15 ml) sesame oil

2 cups plus 1 tablespoon (490 ml) water

1 teaspoon (3.7 g) whole black mustard seeds

1 teaspoon (2.1 g) whole cumin seeds

1 teaspoon (2 g) whole fennel seeds

1 cup (195 g) basmati rice

salt, pinch

lemon, squeeze

Preheat the oven to 375°F (190°C). Place all chopped vegetables in a baking dish and drizzle half of the sesame oil over them. Mix thoroughly, and then add one tablespoon (15 ml) of water to the dish and bake for 50 minutes.

Pour the remaining sesame oil into a small pot and add the seeds. Cook on medium-low heat for 5–7 minutes. Look for a light browning of the fennel and cumin seeds, notice a nutty aroma, and listen for small popping sounds to signal the mustard seeds are done. Add the remaining water to the pot and bring to a boil, and then add the basmati rice. Cook for 1 minute on high, and then stir, reduce heat to low, and cover. Cook for 15–20 minutes or until water is absorbed.

Combine the rice and vegetables, and then add a pinch of salt and a squeeze of lemon to taste and stir.

NOTE: The blend of whole seeds used in this spice mix—fennel, cumin, and black mustard—is such a favorite of mine that I keep a jar of it right beside my stove. The rich, nutty aroma of the seeds when they are roasted in ghee is truly a pleasure to my senses. My dear friend and Ayurvedic colleague Jolie introduced me to this blend. She uses it in rice, bean, and vegetable dishes to improve digestion and assimilation.

tips for your type

FIRE: Use coconut oil instead of sesame oil and lime instead of lemon. Do not use black mustard seeds.

MOUNTAIN: Choose quinoa or amaranth instead of basmati rice; use sesame oil, salt, and lemon sparingly, and add black pepper.

feel the love lemon rice

On my second trip to India, I stayed at a surfing ashram, where a small group of young Hare Krishna devotees lived and shared their spiritual practices—chanting, yoga, and surfing. We would rise each morning at four for chanting and ceremonies, then share a yoga practice at sunrise and take a short boat ride down the river to the ocean, where we would surf until peacefully exhausted and hungry.

Hare Krishnas' tradition relies heavily on service to all as a part of their religious expression, and nourishing people with incredibly delicious, vegetarian food is one of their specialties. I have never been as well nourished and satiated as I was when I stayed with them. I believe it is partly because of the love and devotion they put into each meal, along with the heartfelt service they offer to one another and to their guests. I try to embody that spirit in all of my cooking, and I think the love is palpable—or possibly palatable. This recipe is a variation from a small cookbook they created called *Surfer Grinds*.

YIELD · FOUR ½-CUP (ABOUT 115 G) SERVINGS

1 tablespoon (14 g) ghee

3 shallots, diced

½ jalapeño or green chili pepper, seeded and diced

1 tablespoon (8 g) sesame seeds

1 teaspoon (2.1 g) cumin seeds

½ teaspoon (1.9 g) mustard seeds

3¾ cups (884 ml) water

¼ teaspoon (1.7 g) salt

2 cups (360 g) basmati rice

½-inch piece (13 mm) ginger root, grated or 1 teaspoon (1.8 g) ground ginger

½-inch piece (13 mm) turmeric root, grated or 1 teaspoon (2.2 g) ground turmeric

¼ cup (60 ml) lemon juice

⅛ cup (7 g) chopped parsley

In a large saucepan, sauté the shallots and jalapeño in ghee for 5 minutes on medium heat. Add the sesame, cumin, and mustard seeds and cook for a few more minutes until the sesame seeds turn slightly brown and the mustard seeds make a popping sound. Add the water and salt and turn up to high heat until the water boils, then add the rice, ginger, and turmeric. Reduce heat to low and simmer for 15 minutes, covered, then add the lemon juice and parsley and cook for a few more minutes until all of the water is absorbed.

tips for your type

FIRE: Replace mustard seeds with coriander seeds, reduce salt to ⅛ teaspoon, and do not use jalepeño.

MOUNTAIN: Use only a pinch of salt and eat in moderation.

thick and hearty mung bean vegetable soup

Whole green mung beans are slightly harder than the split variety. For the Breeze, it is best to use them in soup, where the extra water content can soften the bean fully. In this recipe the beans cook long enough to make a thick soup base, and kombu helps improve digestion and reduce gas. If you usually experience gas or bloating, you can also add extra ghee to soften and counter the beans' dryness.

YIELD · FOUR 1-CUP (235 ML) SERVINGS

½ cup (99 g) whole green mung beans, soaked in water

1 quart (946 ml) water

1 piece kombu seaweed

½ cup (75 g) chopped carrots

½ cup (100 g) beets

½ cup (60 g) yellow squash

½ cup (35 g) kale

½ cup (45 g) cabbage, any variety

1 tablespoon (7 g) Warm the Breeze spice mix (see page 86)

1 teaspoon (2 g) garam masala spice mix

1 teaspoon (5 g) ghee

splash of apple cider vinegar or squeeze of lemon

½ teaspoon (3.5 g) salt

Soak mung beans overnight and discard the water in the morning. Place beans in a large stockpot with water and kombu and bring to a boil, then reduce heat to medium-low and simmer. Cook for 45 minutes, remove the kombu, and add all other ingredients. Cook uncovered for another 15–20 minutes, stirring occasionally.

tips for your type

FIRE: Replace beets with zucchini and spices with 1 tablespoon Calm the Fire spice mix (see page 86).

MOUNTAIN: Replace squash and beets with red onion and chard; replace Warm the Breeze with Lift the Mountain spice mix (see page 86); and omit ghee.

baked vegetable medley with zesty herb and tahini sauce

When eating simply with the seasons, I experiment to make new, flavorful sauces to add a little zip. Even the most basic vegetables or grains become different and exciting with a new sauce. This one is a nice assortment of the fresh garden herbs ready for harvest in late summer or early fall, but you can play around with it in each season by substituting other herbs you grow or buy at your local farmers' market or neighborhood co-op. Enjoy a little of your own creative energy along with your meal.

YIELD · FOUR 1-CUP (220 G) SERVINGS

1 medium head cauliflower (900 g), chopped into large florets

6–7 medium tricolor carrots (500 g), chopped

3–4 medium purple or gold potatoes (500 g), quartered

FOR TAHINI SAUCE:
2 tablespoons (30 g) tahini

zest of one small lemon

zest of one medium orange

½ lemon, squeezed

½ orange, squeezed

⅓ cup (20 g) chopped parsley, leaves and soft stems

⅛ cup (6 g) chopped chives

⅛ cup (8 g) chopped dill or fennel leaf

pinch of paprika

pinch of black pepper

2 tablespoons (28 ml) liquid aminos

½ cup (120 ml) water

½ teaspoon (3.5 g) maple syrup

2 tablespoons (28 ml) olive oil or sesame oil

Preheat oven to 425°F (218°C) and place all chopped vegetables in a baking dish with a tablespoon of water. Bake for 15 minutes, then pour the sauce over the vegetables and bake for another 15–20 minutes. When finished, the vegetables will still have a small amount of liquid sauce below them, but the tops should be lightly browned.

FOR THE SAUCE: Combine all ingredients in a blender and puree on high for 1 minute.

tips for your type

FIRE: Enjoy as is, unless the heat of the sauce creates discomfort. Then replace chives with cilantro or basil, use an additional ⅛ cup (12 g) fennel, and omit paprika and black pepper.

MOUNTAIN: Use broccoli instead of sweet potatoes and increase paprika and black pepper to ¼ teaspoon.

lightening cleanse & diet

tHE PURPOSE OF THIS DIETARY CLEANSE is to use stimulating, heating, and reducing practices and foods to lighten the body. The foods consumed are light, dry, and heating in nature with predominantly pungent, bitter, and astringent tastes. The vegetarian diet consists of light and astringent whole grains, legumes, light seeds, and abundant vegetables prepared with heating spices. Oils, fats, salt, fruits, and honey are used sparingly. This cleanse is appropriate for an individual with a Mountain constitution or a Mountain imbalance.

The practices for self-care and daily maintenance include stimulating yoga poses, breathing practices, and vigorous exercise to induce sweating. Heat from the sun, dry sauna, steam, or shower is advisable to create movement and dry up excess secretions. Finally, dry massage with raw silk gloves improves circulation and lymphatic movement to help in cleansing. These practices are all lightening and reducing.

DAILY SELF-CARE PRACTICES

Stimulating, heating, lightening, and reducing are the characteristics that best describe the daily practices for the Mountain or those with a Mountain imbalance. Active and energizing breath practices, yoga poses, and exercise keep the abundant fluids of the body moving to assist cleansing. Massage with raw silk gloves, instead of or in addition to oil massage, improves the circulation and counters heaviness or stagnation.

Integrate these practices into your daily routine during the fourth week of the protocol and strive to continue them in everyday living. Make time for stimulating practices every few hours throughout the day, especially if your work requires you to sit and be still for many hours. A five-minute break every few hours to move and breathe will help, but take a twenty-minute break if you can. Plan time in the morning for as many of these practices as possible to counter the heaviness at that time of day.

RAW SILK MASSAGE

Garshana is the practice of dry massage with raw silk gloves. Much like dry brushing, the slightly rough and nubby texture of the raw silk exfoliates the skin, stimulates circulation and movement of lymph, and removes block-ages to energy. The raw silk also creates a stimulating effect on the nervous system and has a lightening effect on the body. Follow the techniques for oil massage (see pages 92 to 96) while wearing the gloves and give yourself a dry, vigorous scrubbing each morning (see "Resources" on page 202 for garshana glove suppliers). If you have no coating on the tongue, you can apply one to two ounces of oil to your skin after the dry massage. If possible, follow oil application with dry heat or a hot shower or steam.

In the evening, give a short massage to the upper body. Use a dry, vigorous massage on the scalp with strong shampooing motions and use just enough oil on the fingertips to massage the face, neck, and shoulders without pulling on the skin. Bend over for this massage and rest your elbows on your thighs or knees to reduce tension in the shoulders. After the massage, use hot towels to compress the areas oiled—opening the pores, relaxing the muscles, and removing the excess oil.

BREATHING PRACTICES

The right nostril breath increases heat in the body. Use it in the morning to counter the cool qualities present or before meals to improve the strength of the digestive fire. The bellows breath is a stimulating practice that removes congestion from the lungs, increases energy, and has an overall effect of clearing the mind. Use it any time of day or night. Start each practice by finding a comfortable position to sit.

right nostril breath

Block off the left nostril with one hand and continue deep belly breaths or the three-part breath (see page 97) for several minutes.

bellows breath

Take a few deep breaths into the belly. (If this is difficult, start with the deep belly breath and three-part breath on page 97.) Consciously inhale and exhale as fully and deeply as you can. Then speed up the rate of your breaths for thirty seconds without sacrificing their depth. The breath is like a bellows that you use to stoke a fire. Create an even breath in and out, increasing the pace so that you are breathing as fast as you can by the end of the one-minute practice.

After the last exhale, pause, keeping the breath expelled. Sit in stillness and notice how you feel. You may notice a calmness or clear mind. You may also notice that you have no need to inhale right away. You have so fully energized the body that it feels safe to relax. When you need to inhale, sip in a little breath and pause, holding the breath in without any strain. Wait until the body calls for more and enjoy the natural stillness between breaths. Breathe only as often and as much—or as little—as needed to feel comfortable for the next few minutes.

EXERCISE

Commit to daily vigorous cardiovascular exercise that induces sweating as your most important practice. Running, biking, hiking, swimming, skiing, jumping rope, and dancing are just a few of the possible options. For some, the duration required to induce sweating may be 15–20 minutes, but others may require 30 minutes or more. Find options that inspire and excite you so that this becomes a fun and permanent practice.

YOGA POSES

A balanced yoga practice should be stimulating, moving, warming, lightening, and energizing. It should include standing postures with long holds to build heat; back-bending postures to lighten and release the upper body; heating inversions, which require exertion; vinyasa or flowing movement; jumping; or shaking. Use the following postures together or separately when time is limited.

Caution: Unsupported or deep back bends and deep forward bends can place undue pressure on herniated or bulging discs or on the vertebrae when osteoporosis is present. To avoid this, focus on lengthening upward with a gentle lift of the heart instead of reaching backward in standing or unsupported backbends. Gentle, supported backbends are fine as long as there is no discomfort. In forward bends, come forward with a flat back to avoid compression.

Forward bending with the head below the level of the heart is contraindicated for those with uncontrolled high blood pressure. To avoid this, bend forward only halfway so that the head and heart are equidistant from the floor.

supported backbend

Backbends open up the chest and the front of the shoulders, clear the channels for breathing, and lighten the body. Roll up a small towel and place it on the floor or your bed. Lie down so that your mid-back (bra line for women) arches over the towel. Relax in this position for several minutes while practicing deep full breaths.

mountain with sun breath

Stand with your feet hip-width apart, toes spread wide, and the inside arch of the feet parallel to each other. Keep the knees slightly bent with the tailbone reaching downward to lengthen the low back area (this action also pulls the lower abdomen in toward the spine). Imagine holding a block or pillow between the upper thighs and give a gentle squeeze to hold it in place. From this position, lengthen the spine and reach upward through the top of your head.

Focus on your deep breath and move your arms overhead as you inhale, then return the arms to your side as you exhale. Continue with deep full breaths and coordinate the arm movements so that each movement takes the same amount of time as your breath. Now add a gentle backbend at the top of the inhalation (just enough to feel the heart area lift). When you exhale, bend forward with a flat back and reach toward the floor. Only come down as far as you can without rounding the spine—put your hands on your upper thighs for support. Inhale and stand up with a flat back, reaching up to Mountain position with your arms overhead at the top of the inhalation as you did before. Continue this until you feel heat building inside.

warrior to lunge

From the Mountain position, take one big step forward. Now bend both knees, drawing the back knee toward the floor. Straighten the back leg as much as possible: This is the Warrior position. Hold for one minute or longer, keeping your toes pointing forward and your torso upright. On an exhalation, bend the back leg, lowering the knee to the ground while keeping the front knee bent: This is a Lunge position. If you feel strong and steady, move between these two positions. Inhale when lifting up, and exhale when coming down. Repeat several rounds and then switch legs.

TIPS FOR SUCCESSFUL DIETARY CLEANSING

These practices are appropriate for day-to-day maintenance for the individual with a Mountain constitution or imbalance. They are particularly important to follow during the fourth week of the protocol, but they must be modified for the final three days of digestive cleansing to avoid vigorous exercise, yoga, or breath practices.

Meals: Choose the amount of food and type of food for each meal based on your digestive fire. If you have coating on the tongue or a lack of appetite, choose lighter options such as soup or konji—or fast instead. Always eat your biggest or heaviest meal at lunchtime and make the other meals lighter. When possible, use the 100 Steps practice (see page 132) after meals. Drink a spicy tea 30 minutes before each meal and take nectar before or after the meal to improve your digestive fire. Always listen to your burp.

Snacks: Try not to snack between meals. Drink herbal tea or hot water if you feel hunger between meals, then snack on dried fruit or vegetable juice if necessary.

Water intake: Drink warm water with lemon upon rising, then sip on hot water or herbal tea throughout the day to improve the lymphatic circulation. Drink water at appropriate times so that it does not dull the digestive fire—one hour before or two hours after a meal.

Rest: Try to be in bed by 10:30 p.m. so that you can be asleep by 11 p.m. Sleep for only five to six hours; too much sleep can make a Mountain heavy and lethargic. If you are an early sleeper, rise at 4 a.m. for your morning practices. Avoid napping in the daytime and break up sedentary periods of the day with activity when possible.

Self-care: Prioritize the morning time for self-care, including as many practices as possible. Make vigorous exercise the most important practice in your day. If possible, try to stay warm and sweat every day. Avoid too much stillness and take breaks throughout the day to practice stimulating and heating breath practices or yoga poses. Use oil on the body only when the tongue is free of excess coating.

Stress reduction: Use vigorous exercise, stimulating breath, and heating yoga poses to reduce stress.

100 STEPS FOR DIGESTION

To improve digestion, Dr. Vasant Lad, Founder of The Ayurvedic Institute, recommends a gentle walk of approximately one hundred steps after a meal. This practice could be done in conjunction with or in place of a digestive nap (see page 88). For the Mountain, this practice is better because napping in the daytime can increase heaviness.

daily schedule

5–6 a.m.	Wake, ideally after six hours of sleep.
	Drink warm water.
	Eliminate waste from the bowels and bladder.
	Do vigorous exercise, stimulating breath, and/or yoga poses.
	Clean the senses; observe the tongue.
	Do raw silk massage, potentially with a light layer of oil, and take a hot shower or sauna.
7:30 a.m.	Drink tea.
8 a.m.	Breakfast or fast, depending on your appetite.
10 or 11 a.m.	Self-care break with yoga poses or stimulating breath, followed by water intake.
Noon	Drink tea.
12:30 p.m.	Lunch, followed by 100 steps (see sidebar, above).
4 p.m.	Self-care break with yoga poses or stimulating breath, followed by water intake.
5:30 p.m.	Drink tea.
6 p.m.	Light dinner or konji, depending on your appetite.
9 p.m.	Drink warm water or tea if you are hungry (liquids only).
10 p.m.	Do a dry scalp massage, followed by a face, neck, and shoulder massage with light oil and a hot compress afterward.
10:30 p.m.	To prepare for bedtime, roll up a small towel and place it under your mid-back to create a supported backbend; rest for 10–15 minutes in this position; and go to sleep by 11 p.m.

"EAT MORE" LIST
— *for the mountain's daily diet*
and the lightening cleanse —

Choose foods that are **light, dry, and warm** and tastes that are **bitter, astringent, and pungent**.

Eat more of the following:

÷ **fruits** that are dried or astringent in taste, such as apples, apricots, berries, cherries, cranberries, figs, mangoes, peaches, pears, persimmons, pomegranates, prunes, raisins, and, in moderation, lemons

÷ **vegetables** that are bitter, astringent, or pungent, such as asparagus, artichokes, green beans, beets, bell peppers, broccoli, Brussels sprouts, burdock root, cabbage, carrots, cauliflower, celery, chili peppers, cilantro, corn, dandelion greens, daikon, eggplant, garlic, leafy greens, salad greens, onions, parsley, peas, potatoes (white, red, or gold), radishes, spinach, sprouts, winter squashes, turnips, and cooked tomatoes

÷ **grains** that are light, dry, or astringent, such as amaranth, barley, buckwheat, corn, granola, millet, quinoa, and rye

÷ **legumes** of all varieties

÷ **nuts and seeds** that are light, bitter, or astringent, such as pumpkin, flax, and sunflower seeds

÷ **condiments** that are pungent, such as basil, chili peppers, horseradish (wasabi), parsley, scallions, and, in moderation, seaweed

÷ **spices** in abundance, especially ones that are heating and astringent, such as black pepper, cinnamon, cayenne, cloves, garlic, ginger, hing, mustard seed, paprika, turmeric—and, in moderation, cardamom, coriander, cumin, and nutmeg

Use the following sparingly:

÷ **ghee** for cooking

÷ **sweeteners** such as honey or home-grown stevia (see sidebar on page 38)

÷ **oils** of corn, safflower, sunflower, or sesame

Limit or avoid foods that are heavy, dense, slimy, and oily; and tastes that are sweet, sour, and salty

lightening recipes

Most of the recipes are for warm, well-cooked foods and heating spices to kindle a dull digestive fire and improve digestion, assimilation, and elimination. The ingredients are light, dry, and heating, to counter excess Mountain qualities of heavy, moist, and cold. The spice mixes, teas, and recipes include a blend of calming and stimulating foods and spices, to keep circulation moving and counter stagnation while creating a calm but activated mind. Pungent, bitter, and astringent tastes also help the body break down old accumulations. These recipes can be part of a seasonal diet in the spring, year-round for those with a Mountain constitution or imbalance, or during the lightening dietary cleanse.

elevate me tea

Stimulating, bitter, spicy, and exotic, this tea will lift your senses with the smell, the taste, and the tingling it creates inside. Peppermint is a gentle digestive stimulant with a mild warming action that feels cool and tingly. It can relieve indigestion, gas, nausea, stomachache, headache, nervous tension, and insomnia. It can also lift or elevate the mind and emotions as it relieves tension in muscles. This is a great midday pick-me-up when your energy starts to dip!

YIELD · FOUR 1-CUP (235 ML) SERVINGS

1½ tablespoons (4.2 g) dried peppermint

1 tablespoon (8 g) ginger root, grated

2 teaspoons (1 g) dried nettles

1 star anise

1 quart (946 ml) hot water

Fresh mint to garnish

Combine all of the herbs in a large mesh strainer or tea ball and pour boiling water over the herbs into a thermos. Steep 10 minutes, remove the tea ball, and cover to retain the heat. To serve, pour into mugs and garnish with fresh mint leaves.

tips for your type

FIRE: Drink in moderation.

MOUNTAIN: Reduce the ginger root to 1 teaspoon (2.7 g) and drink in moderation.

mountain spice tea

When I am feeling cold and need to reboot my internal fire, this is the tea I choose. It does a wonderful job of building your internal fire to digest food well, burn up toxins, or fight off the latest "bug" going around the school or office. When cleansing, it is great to make a big batch of it in the morning and sip on it throughout the day, given that warming fluids help the lymphatic system—our "internal plumbing"—to drain.

YIELD · FOUR ½-CUP (ABOUT 115 G) SERVINGS

1 tablespoon (8 g) ginger root, grated

6 whole black peppercorns

6 whole green cardamom pods

1 whole clove

1 quart (946 ml) hot water

honey to taste

Combine all ingredients except honey in a large tea ball or fine metal mesh strainer and place in a thermos. Boil water and pour over the strainer into the thermos and cover. Steep the tea for 10–15 minutes and remove the strainer. Remember to pour tea into cups and cool for a few minutes before adding honey (see note, page 87).

tips for your type

BREEZE: To make the tea less heating, cut the ginger root, black pepper, and cardamom in half, leave out the clove, and sweeten with 1 tablespoon of jaggery, a mineral-rich sugar with a molasses-like flavor commonly used in Indian sweets. But you may not want to purchase it straight from India—I'm told it can sometimes contain maggots. Instead, you can purchase organic jaggery from Pure Foods, a company based in New Jersey. Or, you can sweeten with raw or whole cane sugar.

FIRE: This one is too heating for the Fire types, except in times of high ama with a thick, white tongue coating. Then you can make this tea with the modifications for the Breeze.

spring into health juice

Fresh vegetable juice is a popular modern trend in diets and cleansing that classic Ayurvedic texts do not address, because the equipment used to process juice from vegetables was not around 5,000 years ago. Fresh vegetables and fruits have a great deal of prana, and the juice from them therefore carries the same potent energy in concentrated form. In general, juice is cold and raw, so it would better in a warm season or climate—or when the digestive fire is strong. This juice includes the strong pungent taste of ginger, watercress, and daikon radish to counter the natural cooling qualities of fresh juice. The bitter, astringent, and pungent tastes combined in this juice are all good for the Mountain, as they encourage the breakdown of tissues and accumulations. For the Mountain, a fresh glass of juice can be a great midday snack to relieve hunger or cravings for sweets.

YIELD · FOUR 1-CUP (235 ML) SERVINGS

½-inch piece (12.5 mm) ginger root

½-inch piece (12.5 mm) turmeric root

1 cup (60 g) parsley, stems and leaves

1 cup (30 g) watercress or spinach

10 large kale stems

10 celery stalks

1 small golden beet

1 small Chioggia beet

1 small daikon radish

1 green apple

½ head romaine lettuce

½ cup (120 ml) pineapple or pomegranate juice

lemon or grapefruit wedge for garnish

Wash all vegetables and fruits, cut off the inedible stems or tops, and chop into pieces small enough for your juicer. Remove the apple core to prevent the seeds from being juiced, because they contain small amounts of a cyanide compound. Juice and serve with a garnish of lemon or grapefruit.

tips for your type

BREEZE: Replace watercress/spinach and daikon radish with 2 medium carrots and 1 extra apple or beet to make the juice sweeter. Drink occasionally and only in a warm climate or season.

FIRE: Replace ginger, daikon radish, and beets with 1 red apple and 2 medium carrots to reduce the heat of this juice.

tips for your type

BREEZE: Add 3 soaked, pitted dates and 1 tablespoon of ghee to the millet while cooking. Add one soaked, pitted date to the sauce while cooking. Use millet only occasionally, as it is a dry, light, and rough grain.

FIRE: Add 3 soaked, pitted dates, and 1 tablespoon of coconut oil or coconut butter to the millet while cooking. Add one soaked, pitted date to the sauce while cooking.

cinnamon millet porridge with apricot cherry sauce

During spring, the cold and moist qualities of the waning winter season have me wanting a warm, nourishing breakfast, but the melting accumulations inside me would rather I limit heavy, mucus-producing foods. Millet is a dry, astringent grain that can satisfy a strong appetite but leave you feeling light and energized. Warm, sweet cinnamon is also astringent and bitter, helping to dry up excess accumulations in the body as it aids digestion. The mildly sweet apricots and cherries make a tangy sauce for the porridge—no need to add sweetener.

YIELD · FOUR 1-CUP (235 ML) SERVINGS OF PORRIDGE; 1¼ CUPS (ABOUT 300 ML) SAUCE

1 quart (946 ml) water

1 cup (140 g) millet, uncooked

2 teaspoons Sweet Milk spice (see page 86) or 1 tablespoon Spiced honey (see page 86)

pinch of salt

squeeze of lemon

1 cup (246 ml) nut milk or grain milk

spiced honey, if more sweet is desired

FOR SAUCE:

1 cup (130 g) unsweetened, dried cherries (or fresh pitted cherries when available)

½ cup (70 g) dried apricots (or fresh pitted apricots when available)

1½ cups (355 ml) water

¼ teaspoon ground paprika

½ teaspoon (1 g) ground cinnamon

Place 3 cups (706 ml) water in a medium saucepan on high heat and bring to a boil. Add millet, Sweet Milk spice, salt, and lemon and stir together, then reduce heat to low and simmer for 20–25 minutes or until all of the water is absorbed. Place the cooked millet in a blender with the remaining one cup (240 ml) of water and milk, and carefully blend until creamy and smooth. The porridge should pour out of the blender; if not, add more water and blend again.

CAUTION: Leave the blender lid ajar or remove the center insert when blending hot items. The heat will create expansion and pressure inside the blender and could cause the lid to pop off while blending. You can also blend smaller portions to ensure your safety.

FOR THE SAUCE: Combine all ingredients into a small saucepan and cook on medium heat for 15 minutes or until the fruits are mushy and most of the water has been absorbed. Transfer to a blender and mix on low until it makes a chunky sauce. For a thicker sauce, cook until all of the water is absorbed.

To serve, pour the porridge into bowls and place a few tablespoons of sauce on top, then gently swirl the two together. Serve with milk and spiced honey (see page 87) if more sweetness is desired.

NOTE: You can refrigerate the additional sauce or spread and use it another morning on porridge or grits. You can also use it like a chutney with kitchari. When made into a thicker spread, it is a perfect topping for a snack of Gingery Oatmeal Squares (see page 108).

roasted poblano stuffed with chickpeas and spinach

Chickpeas, also called garbanzo beans and many other names, are one of the largest beans, with a slightly dry and rough texture. An abundance of heating and carminative (gas-expelling) spices can improve digestion and eliminate the production of gas that is common with these beans. Soaking the beans overnight—combined with a long, slow cooking process and the addition of kombu—will make them easier to digest. Enjoy the chickpeas alone as a stew or stuffed in a roasted poblano pepper with spinach for more heat and flavor.

YIELD · FOUR 1-CUP (129 G) SERVINGS OVER A ROASTED POBLANO PEPPER WITH ¼ CUP (7.5 G) SPINACH

1 cup (170 g) chickpeas, soaked overnight

water, enough to cover chickpeas by 2 inches (5 cm)

2 strips of kombu

½ cup (75 g) chopped green bell pepper

½ cup (90 g) chopped tomatoes

¼ cup (60 ml) papaya juice

⅛ cup (30 ml) pomegranate juice

1 tablespoon (6 g) ground coriander

1 tablespoon (7.5 g) chili powder

2 bay leaves

1 teaspoon (1.8 g) ground ginger

½ teaspoon (1.2 g) ground cumin

½ teaspoon (2.3 g) black salt

½ teaspoon (1 g) ground black pepper

½ teaspoon (2.7 g) ground fenugreek

¼ teaspoon red pepper flakes

¼ teaspoon ground nutmeg

¼ teaspoon ground cinnamon

¼ teaspoon ground cardamom

TO SERVE:

4 roasted poblano peppers

1 cup (30 g) spinach

Soak chickpeas overnight and discard the water in the morning. Place them in a large stockpot or pressure cooker with all of the ingredients for the chickpeas and then cover with at least 2 inches (5 cm) of water. Bring to a boil and then reduce heat and cover. When using a pressure cooker, secure the lid first and bring up to temperature, then reduce heat to low. Cook for 1–2 hours on low heat until the chickpeas are soft (less time in the pressure cooker). Remove the strips of kombu. (Their role was to add more nutrition and make the beans easier to digest, but they are a little too slimy for most palates.)

Cut the poblano peppers in half and remove the seeds. Place in an oven-safe baking dish and bake uncovered at 425°F (218°C) for 15–20 minutes or until the edges of the pepper brown without burning.

TO SERVE: Place one pepper on a plate, cover with ¼ cup (7.5 g) spinach, and top with 1 cup (129 g) spiced chickpeas.

tips for your type

BREEZE: Reduce chili powder to 1 teaspoon (2.5 g), eliminate red pepper flakes, and add 1 tablespoon (14 g) of ghee while cooking.

FIRE: Reduce chili powder to 1 teaspoon (2.5 g) and eliminate ginger, black pepper, and red pepper flakes. Eat as a stew without the poblano pepper or over a bed of greens.

add it! For non-cleansing meals, add a spoonful of goat cheese and place it between the roasted pepper and the spinach so that it melts with the warmth of the chickpeas on top.

savory corn grits with spicy kale

The foods of south Louisiana are pleasure to the senses—creamy, rich, and spicy—but they do not make for a trim waistline. I set out to make Cajun foods healthy with a little help from Ayurveda (and my Cajun husband). I added more bitter, green vegetables, used ghee instead of butter or lard, and incorporated lighter grains. It was a great success!

YIELD · FOUR 1-CUP (235 ML) SERVINGS

1 quart (946 ml) water

pinch of salt

1 cup (140 g) cornmeal

1 teaspoon (5 ml) sesame oil

1 teaspoon (2.6 g) chili powder

¼ teaspoon ground black pepper

¼ teaspoon ground cayenne pepper

FOR SPICY KALE:

2 cups (135 g) chopped kale

2 cups (135 g) chopped rainbow chard

½ cup (75 g) chopped bell pepper (yellow, orange, or red)

4 cloves garlic, peeled and finely chopped

1 teaspoon (2.7 g) ginger root, grated

1 teaspoon (5 ml) umeboshi vinegar or apple cider vinegar

1 teaspoon (5 ml) toasted sesame oil

¼ teaspoon ground paprika

¼ teaspoon ground black pepper

Place water and salt into a large 2-quart (2 L) saucepan or stockpot and bring to a boil on high heat. Slowly stir in the cornmeal and reduce heat to low. Continue cooking for 20–30 minutes, stirring every few minutes to avoid burning the bottom of the grits or creating firm chunks—the longer the cooking time, the softer and creamier the end result. In the last few minutes of cooking, add 1 teaspoon (5 ml) of sesame oil and all spices, including the nutritional yeast. Remove from heat and serve.

For the spicy kale, combine all ingredients with the remaining ½ teaspoon (2.5 ml) of sesame oil in a large skillet or wok and sauté, covered, for 8–10 minutes on medium heat until all of the water evaporates and the kale is wilted but not shapeless. Serve the corn grits like porridge in bowls and top with spicy kale.

tips for your type

BREEZE: For the grits, use half the amount of spices, ½ teaspoon (3.5 g) of salt, and 2 tablespoons (28 g) of ghee instead of sesame oil. For the spicy kale, use half the amount of spices, including ginger and garlic, 1 tablespoon (14 g) ghee instead of sesame oil, and cook for 5 minutes longer to make the kale softer and easier to digest. You can also use a softer vegetable like zucchini or peas in place of some or all of the leafy greens, which are rough in nature.

FIRE: Omit all of the spices, ginger, garlic, and vinegar. Use ghee instead of sesame oil and add a squeeze of lime.

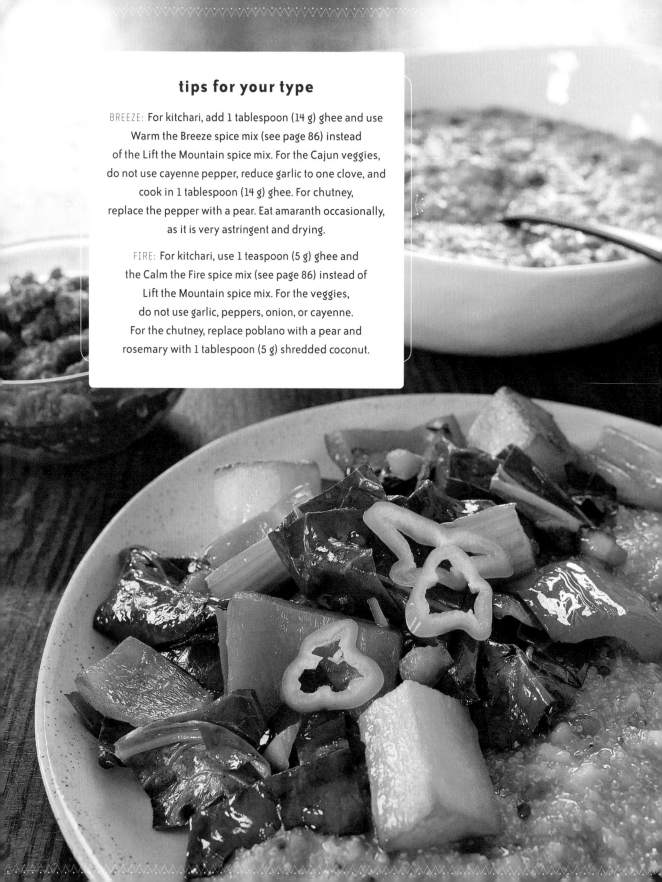

tips for your type

BREEZE: For kitchari, add 1 tablespoon (14 g) ghee and use
Warm the Breeze spice mix (see page 86) instead
of the Lift the Mountain spice mix. For the Cajun veggies,
do not use cayenne pepper, reduce garlic to one clove, and
cook in 1 tablespoon (14 g) ghee. For chutney,
replace the pepper with a pear. Eat amaranth occasionally,
as it is very astringent and drying.

FIRE: For kitchari, use 1 teaspoon (5 g) ghee and
the Calm the Fire spice mix (see page 86) instead of
Lift the Mountain spice mix. For the veggies,
do not use garlic, peppers, onion, or cayenne.
For the chutney, replace poblano with a pear and
rosemary with 1 tablespoon (5 g) shredded coconut.

amaranth kitchari with cajun veggies and cranberry pepper chutney

This version of kitchari is pungent and drying and will give the cool and moist qualities of the Mountain a gentle push toward balance. Amaranth is an astringent grain I like to use in the spring or whenever I feel heavy or congested. You can also use the one-pot cooking method to make this recipe, to improve digestion and reduce preparation time in the kitchen.

YIELD · FOUR 1-CUP SERVINGS KITCHARI AND VEGETABLES (221 G); 1½ CUPS (375 G) CHUTNEY

1 cup (184 g) split green mung beans, uncooked

1 cup (140 g) amaranth, uncooked

1 quart (946 ml) water

1 tablespoon (7 g) Lift the Mountain spice mix (see page 86)

FOR CAJUN VEGGIES:

½ cup (80 g) diced yellow onion

1 cup (120 g) diced celery

3 cloves of garlic, diced

¼ cup (25 g) chopped green onion

1 cup (90 g) chopped purple cabbage

1 cup (140 g) chopped turnips or rutabaga

1 cup (70 g) chopped collard greens

½ teaspoon (2.5 g) ghee or mustard oil

sprinkle of cayenne pepper

pinch of salt

FOR CHUTNEY:

½ cup (65 g) dried cranberries

½ cup (120 ml) water

½ poblano or Anaheim pepper, diced

1 date, soaked overnight in water and pitted

½ teaspoon (1.3 g) cumin seed

¼ teaspoon chopped rosemary

¼ teaspoon grapefruit zest

Rinse mung beans several times and pour off the water to clean any debris from the beans. Combine the beans, amaranth, and water in a large saucepan, then soak overnight. Cook the kitchari (mung beans and rice mixture) with Mountain spice mix on medium-low heat for 30–35 minutes or until the beans are soft and all of the water is absorbed.

Place all ingredients for the Cajun vegetables in a medium sauté pan and cook on medium heat for 25 minutes, stirring occasionally or until the cabbage and turnip/rutabaga are softened but still firm. Serve the vegetables over a bowl of kitchari with cranberry pepper chutney.

FOR CHUTNEY: Place all chutney ingredients except the grapefruit zest in a small saucepan and cook on medium-low until all of the water evaporates (approximately 10 minutes). Add grapefruit zest and transfer to a blender or food processor and mix on low for 30 seconds to 1 minute. The chutney will be blended but will still have some chunks.

tips for your type

BREEZE: Use sweeter salad greens like red or green leaf lettuce—or steam the greens. Eat only in a warmer climate or season, with plenty of oil or dressing.

FIRE: Limit radishes as they are heating. For the dressing, use only ½ teaspoon (1.5 g) garlic, sunflower oil instead of sesame oil, and no black pepper.

grilled vegetables with spring bitters salad and sesame garlic dressing

The first precious little green plants that sprout in the spring are the perfect food-medicine Mother Nature provides to cleanse the body of accumulations from the winter season. These plants are bitter, astringent, and pungent in taste, and vary with climate and geography. Learning where and when to wild-harvest these plants can be a fun and exciting way to connect with nature, as well as with friends and family. In my experience, children love a "pick and eat" adventure hike and are quick to learn which plants to harvest. Look out for ramps, sorrel, nettles, fiddlehead ferns, garlic mustard greens, dandelion greens, and watercress in the wild—or plant radishes, peas, kale, spinach, or green onions in your garden.

YIELD · FOUR 1¹/₂-CUP (150 G) SERVINGS OF GRILLED VEGETABLES; FOUR 1-CUP (36 G) SERVINGS OF SALAD GREENS; 1¹/₂ CUPS (311 G) DRESSING

one bundle of asparagus (approximately 30 thin stalks)

1½ cups (90 g) sweet pea pods

6–8 Spanish black radishes (160 g), thinly sliced

1 large red or orange bell pepper

1 teaspoon (5 ml) sesame oil

FOR SALAD:
½ ounce (10 g) dandelion greens

½ ounce (12 g) water cress

2 ounces (55 g) spinach

2 ounces (55 g) baby kale

2 tablespoons (12 g) chopped scallions or green onions

FOR DRESSING:
½ cup (72 g) sesame seeds, soaked

½ cup (72 g) sunflower seeds, soaked

1 tablespoon (8 g) grated or finely chopped turmeric root

1 tablespoon (10 g) grated or finely chopped garlic

½ cup (30 g) chopped parsley

1 large lemon, squeezed

1 tablespoon (15 ml) flaxseed or sesame oil

¼ teaspoon ground black pepper

¼ cup (60 ml) water

1 teaspoon (5 ml) liquid aminos

Coat the vegetables in a light layer of sesame oil and gently massage them by hand to evenly distribute the oil. Place on a cast-iron grill pan on medium-high heat or on an outdoor grill for a few minutes, until the vegetables soften and lightly brown along the grill lines. Turn the vegetables over and cook a few more minutes, then remove from the heat and let cool. Combine the washed and chopped salad greens in a large serving bowl and place the grilled vegetables over the greens. To serve, place 1 packed cup (36 g) of salad greens on a plate, cover with 1½ cups (150 g) of grilled vegetables, and top with 1–2 tablespoons (13–26 g) of dressing.

NOTE: You can also lightly steam the raw greens for easier digestion.

FOR DRESSING: Place all ingredients in blender and puree on high until smooth.

NOTE: I like to make a larger batch of salad dressing and keep it refrigerated, so that I have a variety of flavors to choose from during the week.

lighten up polenta with squash sauce

Cornmeal is dry and light in nature, so it is a natural choice for the Mountain, but it is often cooked with loads of butter, salt, and cheese or served with a heavy mushroom or tomato sauce. Sesame oil and spices add flavor in this recipe without excessive heaviness, and the sauce is made mostly of acorn squash, which has a slightly sweet yet bitter flavor. Served with broccoli rabe or other steamed green vegetables, this completes the palate of important tastes for the Mountain.

YIELD · SIX "PIE-SLICE" SERVINGS OF POLENTA; THREE CUPS (705 ML) OF SAUCE

1 quart (946 ml) water

pinch of salt

1 cup (140 g) cornmeal

1½ teaspoon (7.5 ml) sesame oil

1 teaspoon (2 g) chili powder

¼ teaspoon ground black pepper

¼ teaspoon ground paprika

¼ cup (14 g) nutritional yeast

FOR SAUCE:

1 medium onion, chopped

1 green pepper, deseeded and chopped

2 cups (115 g) seeded, peeled, and chopped acorn or butternut squash

1 cup (235 ml) water

1 large tomato

1 green chili pepper

1 tablespoon (2 g) Herbs de Provence

SERVE WITH:

steamed or blanched broccoli rabe (or other green vegetables)

Place water and salt into a large 2-quart (2 L) saucepan or stockpot and bring to a boil on high heat. Slowly stir in the cornmeal and reduce heat to low. Continue cooking for 20 to 30 minutes, stirring every few minutes to avoid burning the bottom of the polenta or creating firm chunks— the longer the cooking time, the softer and creamier the end result. In the last few minutes of cooking, add 1 teaspoon (5 ml) of sesame oil and all spices, including the nutritional yeast. Remove from heat and pour or spoon into a round pie plate to cool. *continued on page 150 »*

tips for your type

BREEZE: For the polenta, use half of the spices and 2 tablespoons (28 g) of ghee instead of sesame oil. Polenta is dry and rough in nature, so eat only occasionally. You can eat the breakfast slices like pancakes, with maple syrup or Banana-Berry-Delight Sauce (see page 86).

FIRE: Prepare the polenta without any spices except nutritional yeast and salt—and use ghee instead of sesame oil. For the sauce and breakfast slices, see the Breeze recommendations above.

lighten up polenta, continued

The polenta will firm up in the pie plate in 10–15 minutes and can be sliced into six pieces. To speed up the process, place the pie plate in the refrigerator.

FOR THE SAUCE: Sauté the onion and green pepper in the remaining ½ teaspoon sesame oil (2.5 ml) for 5–7 minutes on medium-low heat, then add the remaining ingredients and simmer for 20–30 minutes until all of the vegetables are soft and the sweet spicy smell fills the air. Good sauces need time for all of the flavors to meld together, so you may want to make the sauce the day before and reheat it when cooking the polenta. Transfer half of the sauce into a blender and puree, first on low and then on medium. Combine the chunks and the puree, then spoon the sauce over the polenta slices to serve.

CAUTION: Leave the blender lid ajar or remove the round center insert when blending hot items. The heat will create expansion and pressure inside the blender and could cause the lid to pop off while blending. You can also blend smaller portions to ensure your safety.

NOTE: To make a breakfast polenta cake, refrigerate the extra polenta slices and then rewarm them in a skillet with a small amount of sesame oil. It is a great combination with the Apricot Cherry Sauce (see page 130).

on the go spicy lentil soup

This is my favorite soup to take on the go. I like to make it drinkable, so that I do not have to carry utensils. Garam masala makes it spicy enough to keep my fire burning strong, even when I am busy working or playing. The lentils always satiate me without any heaviness, which is great for the Mountain.

YIELD · SIX 1½-CUP (112 G) SERVINGS

1½ cups (288 g) lentils, dried

1 quart (946 ml) water

⅔ cup (78 g) daikon radish

⅔ cup (100 g) turnip

⅔ cup (78 g) watermelon radish

⅔ cup (70 g) broccoli stems

¼ cup (40 g) red onion

1–2 teaspoons (4 g) garam masala spice mix

½ teaspoon (2.5 ml) sesame oil

½ teaspoon (3 g) salt

Place all ingredients except salt in a stockpot and bring to a boil over high heat. Reduce heat and simmer, covered, for 30 minutes or until the lentils are soft. Transfer half of the soup to a blender and puree on low, then high for 1 minute. Return the puree to the stockpot and mix with the remaining chunky soup.

CAUTION: Leave the blender lid ajar or remove the round center insert when blending hot items. The heat will create expansion and pressure inside the blender and could cause the lid to pop off while blending. You can also blend smaller portions, to ensure your safety.

NOTE: Garam masala is a traditional spice mix, and the potency can vary with each brand or blend. Start with 1 teaspoon (2 g) spice mix and then taste to see if you need more heat.

tips for your type

BREEZE: Substitute carrots and celery root for daikon and turnips, use ½ teaspoon (1 g) garam masala with ½ teaspoon (1 g) Warm the Breeze spice mix (see page 86), and double the amount of oil.

FIRE: Substitute carrots and celery root for daikon and turnips, use Calm the Fire spice mix (see page 86) instead of garam masala, eliminate onion, and replace sesame oil with sunflower oil.

tips for your type

BREEZE: Use sweeter vegetables like carrot and beet to replace the daikon and radish, 1 clove of garlic, and 15 sweet cherry tomatoes instead of a jalapeño or hot pepper.

FIRE: Use carrots and broccoli to replace daikon and radish and cilantro instead of parsley mix. Omit garlic, jalapeño, and onion.

spring secrets vegetable chili

This chili is packed with many of my favorite spring secrets. The first is a small green daikon radish that has a slightly sweeter taste than the larger and more pungent white variety commonly sold in Asian markets. The watermelon radish looks just like a tiny watermelon when sliced, with a light green skin and a bright fuchsia-colored center; it also has a milder taste, similar to a white radish, that is not as sharp as a red radish. Burdock root is a bitter and pungent vegetable often used in cleansing teas. It is a long, straight, and sturdy brown root that has a carrot-like appearance and a white ringed center. Combined with the bright rainbow-colored stems of the leafy chard and the purple cauliflower, this dish is as beautiful as it is nutritious.

YIELD · SIX TO EIGHT 1-CUP (166-125 G) SERVINGS (DEPENDING ON COOKING TIME AND REMAINING LIQUID)

1 cup (250 g) black beans, soaked overnight

1 cup (170 g) pinto beans, soaked overnight

1½ quarts (1.5 L) water

1 piece kombu seaweed

¼ cup (30 g) chopped daikon or white radish

½ cup (30 g) chopped watermelon radish or rutabaga

1 cup (100 g) purple or white cauliflower

¼ cup (35 g) chopped burdock root or turnips

1 cup (67 g) chopped dandelion greens or rainbow chard

½ cup (80 g) chopped red onion

½ cup (75 g) chopped green bell pepper

3 cloves garlic, minced

1 jalapeño or hot pepper, finely chopped

1 teaspoon (2.6 g) chili powder

½ teaspoon (1.3 g) ground paprika

½ cup (30 g) chopped parsley, thyme, green onions, or a mixture of all three

1 teaspoon (5 ml) apple cider vinegar

¼ teaspoon salt

Soak the black and pinto beans in water overnight, then drain and combine with water and kombu. Cook on medium heat until boiling, then reduce heat to medium low and cover. Cook for 2 hours, stirring occasionally. Remove the kombu from the pot and add all remaining ingredients except salt. Continue cooking for another 25–30 minutes and add the salt in the last few minutes of cooking. The beans should be tender without any crunchiness, but the vegetables should retain their form and have a slight firmness. Beans vary in firmness based on their age and storage, so the amount of time necessary to make them tender always varies. If the beans are not done at this point, add another ½ to 1-cup (120–235 ml) water and continue cooking for another 15 minutes.

tantalizing tempeh and stir-fry wrap

Tempeh is a fermented soy product that has a chewy texture. It is often marinated or covered with spices before cooking. It is simple to prepare quickly. I have a ceramic ginger grater that is easy to use and easy to clean. Just rub the ginger, turmeric, or garlic clove across the ceramic plate, then pour water over it to remove the pieces. Rinse with water again and it is clean. In less then two minutes your tempeh is prepared for cooking. The ceramic grater is also wonderful for fresh ginger tea or fresh grated spices like nutmeg or cinnamon.

YIELD · FOUR LARGE WRAPS OR SIX SMALLER WRAPS

10 ounces (283 g) tempeh, sliced into ½-inch-wide strips

1-inch by ½-inch (25 mm by 13 mm) piece ginger root, grated

1-inch by ½-inch (25 mm by 13 mm) piece turmeric root, grated

1 large clove garlic, peeled and grated

1 teaspoon (5 ml) toasted sesame oil

2 teaspoons (10 ml) liquid aminos

½ lemon, squeezed

FOR STIR-FRY:
1 golden beet, peeled and thinly sliced

1 black radish, thinly sliced

½ green bell pepper

10 Brussels sprouts, quartered

1 cup (100 g) chopped broccolini or Romanesco

3 ounces (84 g) baby spinach

¼ cup (60 g) water

FOR THE WRAP:
2 ounces (55 g) sprouts

gluten-free tortilla or wrap

hummus, optional

Place the sliced tempeh strips into a large sauté pan with the remaining ingredients on top of the tempeh. Lightly massage the ingredients into the tempeh with a hand or spoon (the turmeric may temporarily discolor your hand) and marinate 10 minutes. Cook on medium heat for 10 minutes, turning the tempeh frequently. Remove the tempeh and add the water and chopped veggies to the same pan to use the remaining spices. Cook another 10 minutes on medium heat, until the vegetables begin to soften but are still firm and crunchy in texture. Assemble the tempeh, stir-fry, and fresh ingredients in a gluten-free wrap or tortilla.

OPTIONAL: Use a prepared hummus to stick all of the ingredients in the wrap together—or make your own hummus.

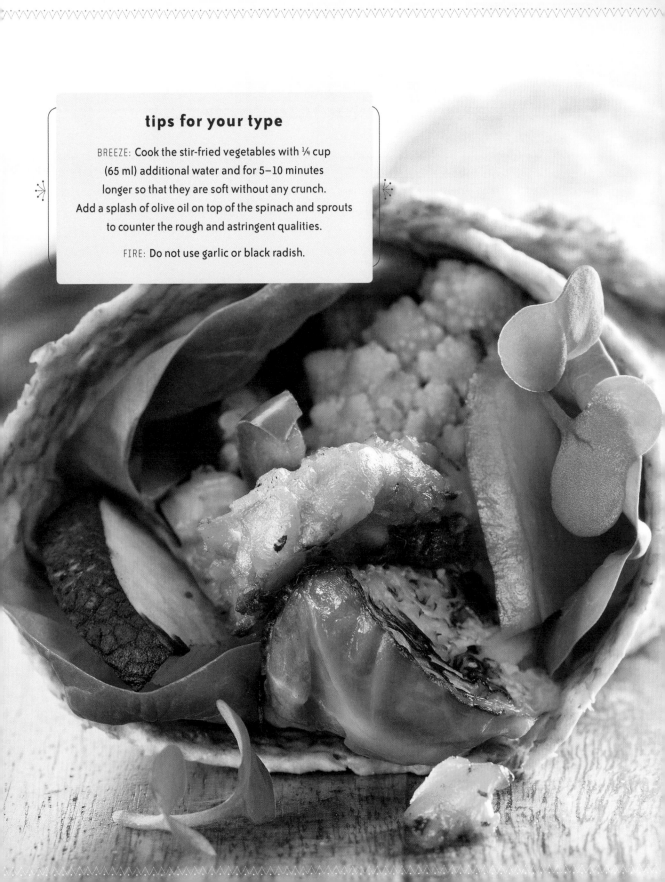

tips for your type

BREEZE: Cook the stir-fried vegetables with ¼ cup (65 ml) additional water and for 5–10 minutes longer so that they are soft without any crunch. Add a splash of olive oil on top of the spinach and sprouts to counter the rough and astringent qualities.

FIRE: Do not use garlic or black radish.

broiled barley with tomato soup

Think creamy tomato soup with herbed croutons—except instead of croutons, you have chewy and slightly crunchy barley. The soup is mostly made of vegetables, with only a small number of tomatoes, as too many sweet, juicy, and moist tomatoes can create a Mountain imbalance. It's comfort food, made healthy!

YIELD · FOUR 1½-CUP (355 ML) SERVINGS

FOR SOUP:

½ cup (50 g) chopped celery

¼ cup (40 g) chopped red onion

½ cup (58 g) chopped daikon or celery root

½ cup (56 g) broccoli stems

1 cup (80 g) chopped bok choy

¼ cup (28 g) chopped fennel

1 cup (180 g) chopped tomato

2 cloves garlic, finely chopped

1 tablespoon (2 g) Herbs de Provence

¼ teaspoon ground black pepper

pinch of salt

2 cups (475 ml) water

FOR BARLEY "CROUTONS":

⅓ cup (65 g) barley, dried

1 cup (235 ml) water

sprinkle of sunflower oil

½ teaspoon (1 g) ground paprika

1 teaspoon (1 g) Herbs de Provence

pinch of salt

FOR GARNISH:

½ cup (30 g) chopped parsley

Place all soup ingredients in a stockpot, bring to a boil on high heat, reduce heat, and simmer for 25 minutes. Once the vegetables are soft, transfer to blender and mix on low for 1 minute for a chunky soup or on high for a creamy soup.

CAUTION: Leave the blender lid ajar or remove the insert when blending hot items. Heat creates pressure in the blender and could cause the lid to pop. Or, blend smaller portions to ensure safety.

In a separate pot, combine water and barley. Bring to a boil on high, then reduce heat, cover, and simmer for 10–15 minutes or until the water is absorbed. Place the cooked barley on a baking sheet and top with the remaining ingredients. Mix to coat evenly, then broil in the oven for 8–10 minutes or until the barley browns slightly.

TO SERVE: Ladle soup into bowls and garnish with broiled barley and chopped parsley.

tips for your type

BREEZE: Use half the amount of paprika and black pepper and substitute oat milk for half of the water in the soup.

FIRE: Eliminate the paprika, black pepper, garlic, and onions, and substitute oat milk for half of the water in the soup.

love my morning soup

The concept of vegetables in the morning was unfamiliar to me before I studied yoga and Ayurveda. I am grateful to the kitchen of the Kripalu Yoga Center, in Stockbridge, Massachusetts, for the kind introduction. For years they put out a steaming pot of simple vegetable soup every morning, with options to add grains, spices, or miso to your liking. I found that it changed the way I felt in the morning, from heavy to light and refreshed. I like to pack in the vegetables and start the day with a giant dose of greens when I make this soup. I always feel light but nourished with this breakfast—I love my morning soup!

YIELD · SIX 1-CUP (235 ML) SERVINGS

1 quart (946 ml) water

1 tablespoon (3 g) dulse flakes

3 cups (200 g) torn or chopped kale, in one-inch square pieces

1 cup (80 g) chopped broccoli, in spoon-sized bites

1 onion or leek, chopped

¼ cup (55 g) chopped red beet, in thinly sliced quarters

¼ cup (43 g) quinoa, uncooked

1 clove garlic, diced or grated

1-inch piece ginger root, grated

miso paste (optional, to taste)

Place all ingredients in a medium to large stockpot, bring to a boil on high heat, then reduce heat to medium and simmer uncovered for 30–35 minutes. Serve in bowls and stir in ½ teaspoon (3 g) of miso paste per cup of soup if desired.

NOTE: Miso is a fermented grain or legume paste traditional to Japanese cooking. It is salty and sour. It is available in many varieties and is an easy way to add flavor to soup or sauces. Chickpea miso is light in color and flavor and is great for sauces or soups in a warmer season. Barley miso has a deep, rich, earthy flavor that makes a thick soup for cold winter mornings. Brown rice miso is also hearty and full in flavor, with a softer feel. Red pepper miso is my favorite, with a little heat and a little sweet. A little goes a long way, so use sparingly—especially if you have a Mountain or Fire imbalance.

tips for your type

BREEZE: Use ½-cup (95 g) short-grain brown rice instead of quinoa and replace half of the kale with 1 cup (130 g) chopped carrots.

FIRE: Use 1 cup (100 g) cauliflower in place of the onion and garlic. Eat miso only occasionally, because it is salty and fermented.

cooling cleanse & diet

tHE PURPOSE OF THIS DIETARY CLEANSE is to lighten the body with a vegetarian diet of cooling foods and practices that reduce heat and accumulations. The diet consists of whole grains, legumes, nuts and seeds, fresh fruits and vegetables, cold-pressed oils and ghee, spices, and natural sweeteners that are all cooling in nature. These foods are predominantly sweet, bitter, and astringent in taste and are appropriate for those with a Fire constitution or imbalance.

These daily practices and self-care techniques are designed to be cooling, calming to the nervous system, and rejuvenating for the mind. The yoga poses, breathing practices, and exercise choices described aim to reduce Fire imbalances. Daily oil massage focuses on the head and feet and is applied with cooling oils in a gentle, soothing manner.

DAILY SELF-CARE PRACTICES

Actions for self-care of a Fire individual or a person with a Fire imbalance should be cooling, soothing, and calming. Avoid intensity or extremes. The Fire individual is commonly an "all or nothing" person with a strong drive for doing. Cultivating a middle-of-the-road mentality for this fourth week, and ideally for the rest of life, is important to finding balance.

Relaxing massage, breath practices, and yoga in the morning and evening will help set the tone for a day of activity and a night of sleep. Cooling practices in the daytime will counter the accumulation of heat from the season and climate, activity, or mental work. It is advisable to take some time away from a busy or intense work schedule during the week of cleansing or find a way to back off 30 percent from everything.

OIL SELF-MASSAGE

Daily self-massage can be done in the morning or in the evening, whichever time of day allows for more leisure in the massage (see pages 92 to 96 for instructions). If the full-body oil massage is in the morning, do a short head and foot massage at night before bedtime.

BREATHING PRACTICES

You can use the deep belly breath or three-part breath (see page 97) in the morning and evening to create relaxation, and the cooling breath during the daytime. It is helpful to take regular self-care breaks to practice this breath (followed by water intake) or to use it when emotions flare up. You can use both breath practices in a reclining or seated position.

cooling breath

Curl the sides of the tongue up to create a small channel and sip air in as if sipping through a straw. Feel the cool air move across the soft and hard palate as you inhale. This air passes across the tiny blood vessels that nourish the brain, relaying a cooling effect physically and emotionally. Exhale through the nostrils and continue this breath for several minutes or until you feel cooled and calmed.

YOGA POSES

Key words in a balancing yoga practice for a Fire individual are cooling, relaxing, surrendering, soothing, and gentle. An attitude of forgiveness and compassion for oneself and others is a good focus for yoga on and off the mat. Postures that open or wring out the middle region of the torso help release accumulated heat and toxins from the digestive organs. Twists, seated postures, cooling inversions, standing postures with wide legs, and forward bends are all appropriate. Childlike free-flowing movements are also helpful. Try these postures for their cooling effects.

Precautions: Inversions when the heart is higher than the head are contraindicated for individuals with uncontrolled high bold pressure; however an inversion of the legs (see right) with the head and the heart at the same level is fine.

Twists may cause undue strain on herniated or bulging discs in the spine, depending on the location of the injury. Use caution and move slowly so that you can stop if you feel pain or discomfort.

twist

Sit in a comfortable position with both legs extended. Use cushions, folded blankets, or blocks under your hips so that you can sit without strain in the low back. Bend your left leg, cross it over your straight right leg, and place the sole of the foot on the floor near your right knee. Sit here and take deep belly breaths. Using your core strength, rotate your torso left and let your right hand rest on your left knee. Place your left hand behind you on the floor for support. Now breathe deeply and try to relax the belly and expand the rib cage. Stay here for several breaths and then slowly release. Switch legs and repeat.

inversion—legs up the wall

Find a place along a wall where you can relax in a lying position with your straight legs extended toward the

twist

inversion—legs up the wall

ceiling. Rest your legs on the wall and make yourself as comfortable as possible, with pillows or blankets for support. Cover the eyes and relax with deep belly breaths for 5–10 minutes. If you do not have a space along a wall, lie on the floor with knees bent at a 90-degree angle and rest your lower legs on a sofa or bed.

EXERCISE

Activities and exercise in nature are helpful for balancing the Fire individual. Nature itself has a calming effect on the Fire, and the cooling attributes of water enhance this. Swimming or walking near water is an ideal form of exercise, but any activity that is noncompetitive, leisurely, or playful is appropriate. To find balance, avoid exercise outdoors in the heat of the day and exercise that is intense or strenuous. Exercising in the cooler morning hours is advised.

TIPS FOR SUCCESSFUL DIETARY CLEANSING

These suggestions are helpful on a daily basis for those with a Fire constitution or imbalance, but are an essential part of the fourth week of the protocol. For the final three days of digestive cleansing, modify these recommendations to avoid cold foods and exercise.

Meals: Drink cooling teas before or with a meal and take nectar with breakfast and dinner only (if your fire imbalance is strong, avoid nectar altogether). Eat enough food to be satiated and, whenever possible, take a digestive nap or use the 100 Steps practice after each meal.

Snacks: Snack on fresh fruit, vegetable juice, nut milks, or konji, but when hunger appears, always drink water; the desire for water is often mistaken as hunger.

Water: Drink warm water upon rising, then drink room temperature water throughout the day and avoid any drinks colder than that. Drink only a small amount of water with meals. Take self-care breaks to drink water between meals.

Rest: Try to be in bed without stimulation by 9:30 p.m., so that you can be asleep before 10 p.m. If a second wind arises, you may feel hungry and your sleep may be delayed. If hunger does arise, have a warm-milk drink, and if sleep is delayed, calm the nervous system with self-care practices.

Self-care: You can divide daily practices equally between morning and evening self-care routines. Calming practices should be the priority in the morning and evening and cooling practices during the day. You can do oil massage at any time, but you should do a head and foot massage every evening (even if you had a full-body oil massage in the morning).

Stress reduction: Spend time in nature, particularly around or in water for exercise and to reduce stress. Incorporate breath practices or yoga poses in your self-care breaks to diffuse intensity and heat during the day. Make time for stillness and avoid excessive work or stimulation during the fourth week.

daily schedule

6 a.m.	Wake, ideally after seven hours of sleep.
	Practice deep breaths.
	Practice twists (seated, as pictured on page 161, or lying in bed).
	Drink warm water.
	Eliminate wastes from the bowels and bladder.
	Walk in nature.
	Clean the senses; observe the tongue.
	Oil and shower.
7:30 a.m.	Drink tea or juice.
8 a.m.	Breakfast, followed by 100 steps if a nature walk did not happen earlier (see page 132).
10:30 or 11 a.m.	Self-care break with cooling breath or yoga poses, followed by water intake.
Noon	Drink juice or tea.
12:30 p.m.	Lunch (the biggest and heaviest meal), followed by 100-step walk or a digestive nap (see page 88).
4 p.m.	Self-care break, with cooling breaths, legs up the wall, and water intake.
5:30 p.m.	Drink tea or juice.
6 p.m.	Dinner.
9 p.m.	Practice deep breaths and candle-gazing meditation; oil head and feet, and place oil in ears.
9:30 p.m.	Prepare for bedtime; go to sleep by 10 p.m.

"EAT MORE" LIST
— for the fire's daily diet
and the cooling cleanse —

Choose foods that are **cooling** in nature and tastes that are **sweet, bitter, and astringent**.

Eat more of the following:

÷ **fruits** that are sweet, cooling, or astringent, such as apples, avocadoes, dates, figs, grapes, limes, melons, pears, persimmons, pomegranates, raisins, and watermelon. Consume berries, cherries, oranges, peaches, plums, and pineapples only if they are sweet.

÷ **vegetables** that are green, bitter, and astringent, especially asparagus, broccoli, Brussels sprouts, celery, cucumber, green beans, green peppers, kale, leafy greens, lettuce, parsley, peas, yellow squash, zucchini, and all kinds of sprouts. *Eat in moderation*: carrots, cauliflower, cabbage, okra, potatoes, squash, and white or yellow onions (if well cooked). *Eat occasionally and in season*: fresh corn and fresh and sweet cherry tomatoes (from your garden, if possible)

÷ **grains** that are cooling or astringent, such as amaranth, barley, granola, basmati rice, wild rice, quinoa, oats, wheat

÷ **legumes** of all varieties, including tofu and tempeh

÷ **nut and seeds** that are cooling, such as coconut, almonds, sunflower, and pumpkin seeds

÷ **ghee and raw cow's milk** as a food-medicine for lubrication and nourishment (If you consume dairy; otherwise use soy, almond, or cashew milk.)

÷ **oils** that are cooling, such as coconut, sunflower, safflower, and olive oil (all in moderation, because Fire individuals have a slightly oily quality by nature)

÷ **sweeteners** such as maple syrup, raw sugar, homemade stevia, or whole cane sugar

÷ **condiments** that are cooling, such as cilantro, lime, and mint; rock salt and seaweed in moderation

÷ **spices** that are cooling, sweet, bitter, or astringent, such as cardamom, coriander, cumin, fennel, saffron, turmeric; *eat occasionally*: cinnamon, fresh ginger, and nutmeg

÷ **mushroom broth, bone broths, or meat** of chicken, turkey, or venison (if you eat meat) for **non-cleansing** times or rejuvenation

Limit or avoid foods that are sour, salty, and pungent in taste, especially heating spices, hot peppers, garlic, uncooked onions, and vinegar.

cooling recipes

The following recipes combine cooked and raw foods, with ingredients that are all calming in nature. Abundant green vegetables provide the bitter and astringent tastes that create a natural cleansing action in the body. All recipes involve mostly cooling ingredients, limiting salty, sour, and pungent foods and spices that increase the Fire imbalances. These recipes are good as part of a seasonal diet in the summer, for those with a Fire constitution or imbalance year-round, or as part of the Cooling dietary cleanse.

the cool-down "iced" tea, summer soothe tea, cool as a
cucumber summer cleanse juice (clockwise from left)

the cool-down "iced" tea

A tea made of coriander, cumin, and fennel is an Ayurvedic staple for aiding digestion without increasing the Fire, or heat, in the body. Cooled for summertime, this "iced tea" is better than traditional iced tea because it has no caffeine. Even though it is called "iced tea," serve it at room temperature so that it is easily digested and assimilated. Ayurveda recommends avoiding foods and liquids that are colder than room temperature. It is recommended that you drink the tea warm during the final three days of digestive cleansing.

YIELD · APPROXIMATELY 2 QUARTS (2 L) OF TEA; SIX 12-OUNCE (355 ML) SERVINGS

2 tablespoons (10 g) whole coriander seed

1 tablespoon (6 g) whole cumin seed

1 tablespoon (6 g) whole fennel seed

1–2 teaspoons (3.5–7 g) licorice root or 8 drops homemade liquid stevia

1 quart (946 ml) boiling water

4 cups (946 ml) ice, cubed or crushed

1 lemon, sliced for garnish

Place coriander, cumin, fennel, and licorice in a large mesh strainer or tea ball and place in a thermos. Pour boiling water into the thermos and allow the herbs to steep for 10–15 minutes, then transfer the tea to a pitcher, pouring it over ice to cool. Garnish each glass with a lemon slice to squeeze into the tea.

CAUTION: Anyone who has high blood pressure should not consume licorice root tea. Use homemade liquid stevia (see page 38) to add sweetness as an alternative.

tips for your type

BREEZE: Add 1 teaspoon (3 g) grated ginger to the tea.

MOUNTAIN: Add 1 tablespoon (8 g) grated ginger to the tea and use homemade liquid stevia sparingly.

summer soothe tea

Soothe the internal heat of summer with this cooling drink. Nettles and raspberry leaf are both rich in minerals, cooling, and astringent in nature. Raspberry leaf is better for relieving menstrual complaints while nettles builds the blood with its high iron content. Rose and hibiscus flowers are astringent and sweet, with qualities that cool not only the body but also the mind and emotions. Both flowers are commonly used in devotional practices and are said to work on the blood and heart, physically and spiritually. When I start drinking it in the summer, I crave it every day.

YIELD · APPROXIMATELY 2 QUARTS (2 L); SIX 12-OUNCE (355 ML) SERVINGS

1 tablespoon (2 g) dried nettles or raspberry leaf

1 tablespoon (4 g) dried rose petals

1 teaspoon (2 g) dried hibiscus flowers

1 quart (946 ml) water

8 drops homemade liquid stevia (see sidebar on page 38)

4 cups (946 ml) ice, crushed or cubed

lime for garnish

Combine dried herbs and water in a sealed glass container and place it in the sun for one afternoon. For faster preparation, combine the dried herbs with boiling water in a thermos and steep for 10 minutes. Add stevia and pour into a pitcher over ice to cool. Serve with a garnish of lime to squeeze into each glass.

tips for your type

BREEZE: Add ½ cinnamon stick to the tea blend and drink only in a hot season. Drink in moderation as the astringent nature can be too drying.

MOUNTAIN: Add 1 cinnamon stick to the tea blend, use less stevia, and drink only in a hot season. The astringent nature is wonderful for the Mountain, but to counter the cold nature, this type can drink it warm.

cool as a cucumber summer cleanse juice

This juice contains many of the best pitta-reducing foods. On a hot summer day, it feels like a glass of liquid revitalization. Each food on this list can help reduce internal or external accumulations of heat—apply mashed cilantro to the skin for sunburn or hives and to counter dehydration from sun exposure, drink coconut water. Be aware that the synergistic effect of this bitter and sweet drink is a powerful food-medicine. A daily glass will keep Fire individuals refreshed and energized. I like to finish a long day at the beach with this juice, a cool shower, and a lavender essential oil and coconut oil self-massage, to soothe the inside and the outside.

YIELD · FOUR 1-CUP (235 ML) SERVINGS

6 large kale stems

2 fennel stalks

6 celery stalks

2 large cucumbers

6 romaine lettuce leaves

2 red apples

1 cup (8 g) cilantro, stems and leaves

½ cup (120 g) fresh green coconut water or bottled coconut water

mint sprigs to garnish

½ lime, sliced to garnish

Wash all fruits and vegetables, cut off inedible stems or ends, and chop into pieces. Remove the apple core, as the seeds contain small amounts of a cyanide compound. Juice, mix with coconut water, pour into glasses, and garnish with fresh mint and lime.

NOTE: Young green coconuts have a smooth but hard outer shell, soft internal flesh, and a thin, clear liquid inside that is commonly bottled and sold as coconut water. The immature coconut has a noticeably different flavor from the mature variety. Young coconuts are often available in specialty markets and are fun to try if you have never had the experience. To open, puncture a hole in the shell with a sharp object and pour out the water. Then use a machete or large, sturdy knife to chop open the top of the coconut and scoop out the white or pinkish flesh.

tips for your type

BREEZE: Use half the amount of all listed ingredients and add 3 medium carrots, 2 beets, and a ¼-inch (6mm) piece of ginger to aid digestion.

MOUNTAIN: Use green apples, double the amount of kale and romaine, add one cup of spinach, and replace cucumber and coconut water with 2 large broccoli stems and a ½-inch (13 mm) piece of ginger.

FOR BOTH: Drink occasionally and only in a warm season or climate.

turmeric "latte"

Turmeric is a sweet and bitter root that is great replacement for the bitter of coffee. It can reduce inflammation, enhance proper functioning of the liver, cool the body, and clear out toxins. Warm turmeric milk is a common Ayurvedic recommendation for rejuvenation of the Fire imbalance. Turmeric's underlying effect on the body is calming (sattvic), so you can enjoy the ritual of your warm morning drink without the stimulating effects that bring craving and imbalance later in the day.

YIELD · TWO 1-CUP (235 ML) SERVINGS

2 cups (475 ml) fresh almond milk (see page 104)

½-inch by 1-inch piece (13 mm by 25 mm) turmeric root, grated

1 tablespoon (4 g) dried rose petals

1 teaspoon (1 g) dried chamomile flowers

pinch of nutmeg

pinch of cardamom

1 teaspoon (5 g) ghee

1 date, soaked overnight in water and pitted

Combine all ingredients except the date in a small saucepan and warm on medium-low heat for 10–15 minutes until the mixture comes to a gentle boil. Remove from heat, strain, and pour into the blender. Add the date and blend on low, then high, to create a foamy, frothy head on the milk. Pour into cups and serve.

CAUTION: Leave the blender lid ajar or remove the round center insert when blending hot items. The heat will create expansion and pressure inside the blender and could cause the lid to pop off while blending. You can also blend smaller portions to ensure your safety.

COFFEE

Regular consumption of bitter foods improves the flavor of the other five tastes. Bitter clears the palate and brings discernment to the tongue. Most people do not consume adequate bitter taste in the form of dark, leafy greens, nettles or bitter teas, bitter roots, or other green vegetables, so coffee with its roasted bitter flavor can easily feel like the antidote to that deficiency. Despite its delicious flavor, coffee is hot, sharp, and oily, and can increase these qualities in the body, dehydrate it, tax the liver, and overstimulate the digestive, elimination, and nervous systems.

tips for your type

BREEZE: Add a pinch of ground ginger and
an extra pinch of cardamom.

MOUNTAIN: Add ¼ teaspoon of ground ginger and
cinnamon. Do not add rose, chamomile, ghee, or dates;
sweeten as needed with spiced honey instead.

coconut almond porridge with baked pears and apples

"Cooling, cooling, and more cooling" is the best label for this recipe. When the heat of summer or the imbalance of Fire is flaring, reach for this delicious breakfast recipe anytime of day. It combines two useful tools for slowing down and firming up soft eliminations caused by excessive heat: the first is apples cooked with ghee and cinnamon, and the second is plain basmati rice. The combination of these, along with additional cooling ingredients like coconut, dates, and pears, should be a staple for those with fire on the rise!

YIELD · FOUR ¾-CUP (110 G) SERVINGS

1 cup (180 g) basmati rice, uncooked

¼ cup (21 g) shredded coconut

20 almonds, soaked overnight in water and peeled

1 cup (235 ml) coconut milk

1 teaspoon (2 g) Sweet Milk spice (see page 86)

pinch of mineral salt

3 dates, soaked overnight in water and pitted

3 cups (710 ml) water

FOR BAKED FRUIT:
1 apple, sliced

1 pear, sliced

¼ teaspoon ground cinnamon

1 teaspoon (5 g) ghee

2 teaspoons (10 ml) water

Combine all ingredients with 2 cups (475 ml) of water in a large saucepan and cook on high heat until the water boils. Reduce heat to low, cover, and simmer on low heat for 20 minutes or until the water is absorbed. Transfer to a blender with the remaining 1 cup (235 ml) of hot water and puree first on low, then on high until creamy and smooth. The porridge should be pourable when complete, so add more water if necessary.

CAUTION: Leave the blender lid ajar or remove the round center insert when blending hot items. The heat will create expansion and pressure inside the blender and could cause the lid to pop off while blending. You can also blend smaller portions to ensure your safety.

FOR THE BAKED FRUIT: Place all ingredients in a covered baking dish and bake at 350°F (176°C) for 30–35 minutes. Make sure the apples are soft or even mushy, for easy digestion. Serve the baked fruit on top of the porridge.

tips for your type

BREEZE: Replace coconut milk with oat or nut milk and add ¼ teaspoon of ginger powder to the porridge.

MOUNTAIN: This porridge is too heavy and cooling for the Mountain. Instead, double the apple and pear recipe, add 1 teaspoon (2 g) ginger powder, and eat the baked fruit only.

creamy cauliflower and wild rice soup

Cauliflower makes a delicious, creamy base for soup without any oil or dairy products. Wild rice, which is not truly rice but a long, hearty seed from an aquatic freshwater grass, is full of protein, minerals, and B vitamins. Wild rice expands four-fold when cooked, so a small amount of dry seed will nourish many.

YIELD · FOUR 1½-CUP (353 ML) SERVINGS

3 cups (300 g) cauliflower

2 cups (475 ml) oat milk

2 cups (475 ml) water

½ cup (160 g) wild rice

¾ cup (54 g) chopped broccoli

¾ cup (110 g) peas

1 teaspoon (1 g) Herbs de Provence

mineral salt to taste

Bake cauliflower in the oven at 350°F (176°C) in a covered dish with a few tablespoons of water for 45 minutes or until it is very soft and falls apart on contact. Place in a blender with oat milk and water and puree on low, then high for 1 minute until smooth and creamy. Transfer the cauliflower soup base to a stockpot, add wild rice, and bring to a boil. Reduce heat to low, cover, and simmer for 45 minutes, stirring occasionally. Add the chopped broccoli, peas, and spices and cook for another 15 minutes.

CAUTION: Leave the blender lid ajar or remove the round center insert when blending hot items. The heat will create expansion and pressure inside the blender and could cause the lid to pop off while blending. You can also blend smaller portions to ensure your safety.

tips for your type

BREEZE: Enjoy!

MOUNTAIN: Substitute 2 cups (475 ml) water for oat milk and add ¼ teaspoon black pepper. Eat in moderation.

add it! For times of rejuvenation, substitute two cups (475 ml) mushroom or bone broth (turkey or chicken) for the oat milk.

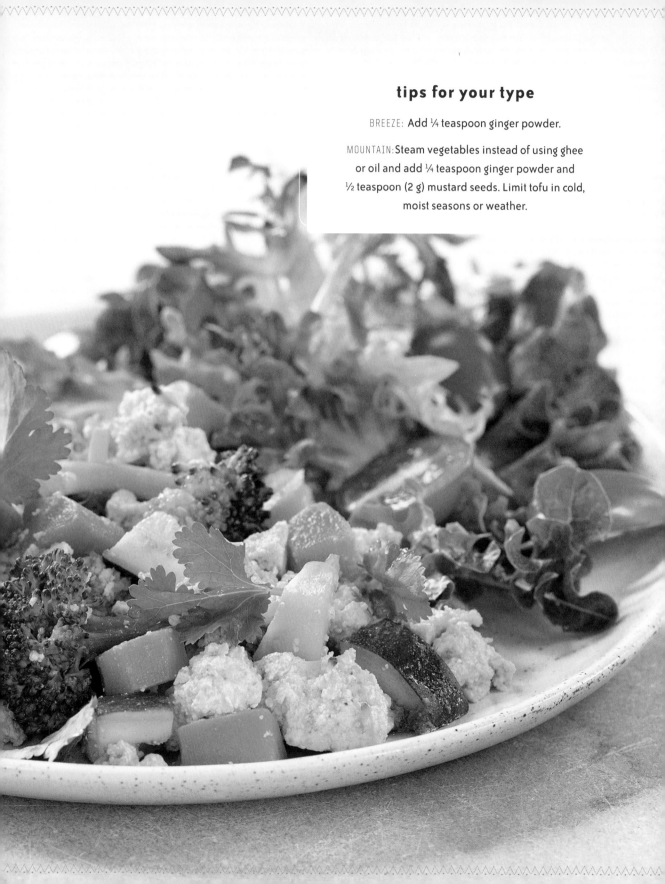

tips for your type

BREEZE: Add ¼ teaspoon ginger powder.

MOUNTAIN: Steam vegetables instead of using ghee or oil and add ¼ teaspoon ginger powder and ½ teaspoon (2 g) mustard seeds. Limit tofu in cold, moist seasons or weather.

"swami's secret" tofu scramble

This recipe is dedicated to the swami who first introduced me to Ayurveda and Sanskrit, the language of traditional yogic and Ayurvedic texts. He excelled at storytelling, chanting, singing, cooking, and laughing. I still hear his deep, bellowing voice in my head every time I chant "Om." I am eternally grateful to him for his knowledge and for the culinary secret to making tofu scramble taste like eggs: "black salt." It is actually pink in color and very fine in texture, with a sulfur-like aroma—and is available at Indian markets. I also like to use nutritional yeast to add a "cheesy" flavor; it is full of B vitamins and ideal to consume with a vegetarian diet to ensure proper nutrition.

YIELD · FOUR 1-CUP (196 G) SERVINGS

15 ounces (420 g) firm tofu, pressed and crumbled

1 cup (71 g) chopped broccoli

1 cup (130 g) chopped carrots

1 cup (120 g) chopped yellow squash or zucchini

1 teaspoon (5 g) ghee or coconut oil

2 tablespoons (30 ml) water

1 tablespoon (15 ml) olive oil

½ teaspoon (1 g) ground cumin

½ teaspoon (1 g) ground fenugreek

½ teaspoon (1 g) ground coriander

1 teaspoon (2 g) ground turmeric

squeeze of lemon or lime

½ teaspoon (2 g) black salt (pink in color and very fine)

splash or capful of apple cider vinegar

1 teaspoon (1 g) nutritional yeast

FOR GARNISH:
1 tablespoon (3 g) chopped basil or cilantro

6–12 sweet cherry tomatoes (only when ripe and in season)

Drain the water from the tofu, slice it into ½-inch (13 mm) thick slabs, and "press" the tofu to remove the excess moisture. Place one clean cloth or towel over a cutting board and arrange the tofu on top of the towel. Then place a second cloth over the tofu and a heavy cookbook on top. Push down firmly and evenly on the cookbook to press the tofu for 1 minute, then leave the book in place for another 10 minutes.

Place the chopped veggies in a sauté pan with ghee or coconut oil and water. Cover with a lid and water-sauté for 15 minutes on medium heat. Push the vegetables to the sides of the pan, place the ghee or oil and spices in the center of the pan, and cook for 1 minute to release the aroma of the spices. Then crumble the slabs of tofu into the pan over the spices and stir together to coat the tofu evenly so that it turns an egg-like color. Add lemon or lime, black salt, and nutritional yeast directly to the tofu, stir gently, then mix in the other vegetables. Cook for a few more minutes to allow the flavors to meld. Garnish with chopped basil or cilantro and a few sweet cherry tomatoes only when fully ripe and in season.

summer sunrise pudding

It is easy to see why chia is so popular. It is a high-protein food with a mild flavor that blends well with anything and has a slippery quality that is good for the digestive tract. This is one super food that is super easy to make into a healthy breakfast—and so delicious it could be dessert. My morning ritual in the summer starts with a sunrise at the beach and a bowl of fresh fruits, nuts, seeds, and coconut milk to keep me cool and nourished. If you don't have the beach, you can still have the sunrise in your bowl.

YIELD · FOUR 1-CUP (235 ML) SERVINGS

¾ cup (175 ml) coconut milk

¾ cup (175 ml) oat milk

¾ cup (102 g) sweet berries

1 mango, sliced

1 cup (115 g) granola (preferably with almonds and pumpkin seeds) or sprouted grains

¼ cup (48 g) chia seed

Fruits and fresh coconut for garnish

Combine coconut milk, oat milk, and ½ cup (75 g) fresh fruit in a blender and puree on high for 1 minute. Pour into a quart-sized (1 L) container with lid and mix in granola or sprouted grains and chia seed. Refrigerate overnight and serve in the morning topped with an assortment of berries, mango, or fresh coconut for garnish. You can also warm the pudding on low heat for a few minutes to counter the refrigerated cold.

tips for your type

BREEZE: Warm the pudding and eat in a warm season.

MOUNTAIN: This breakfast is very sweet, with cold and slippery qualities that are not good for the Mountain. Eat in small portions, only on occasion, and in a warm season.

sweet green goodness soup with cucumber raita

This soup is so creamy and sweet that I made it for my daughter as one of her first solid foods and for a friend receiving cancer treatment when nothing else was palatable. The recipe has had many variations throughout the years, but it remains a cooling, soothing staple for me. This version adds raita, a cooling side dish from traditional Indian cuisine, and a garnish of raw foods.

YIELD · FOUR 1-CUP (235 ML) SERVINGS

2 large zucchini, chopped into 1-inch (2.5 cm) cubes

½ cup (75 g) peas

1 large potatoes, chopped into 1-inch (2.5 cm) cubes

¼ cup (4 g) chopped cilantro, stems and leaves

¼ teaspoon (2 g) salt

1 cup (235 ml) water

1 teaspoon (5 g) ghee

½ lemon or lime, squeezed

FOR RAITA:

1 teaspoon (2 g) whole cumin seed

½ teaspoon (3 g) ghee

½ cup (115 g) unsweetened yogurt

½ cucumber, peeled and diced

1½ tablespoons (6 g) chopped dill

pinch of black pepper

pinch of mineral salt

FOR GARNISH:

5–10 zucchini strips, thinly sliced

pinch of sprouts (alfalfa, sunflower, mung, or pea shoots are all good choices)

1 teaspoon (2 g) ground pumpkin seeds

Combine all ingredients in a medium stockpot, cover with a lid, and cook on medium heat for 20 minutes. At first, the solid chunks of vegetables will not be immersed in the water. Stir every 5 minutes, and as it cooks down, the vegetables will soften and sink into the water. The soup is done when all of the chunks are immersed in the water and soft. Transfer to a blender and puree. If you prefer chunky soup, puree half of the vegetables with all of the liquid and pour over the remaining chunks.

CAUTION: Leave the blender lid ajar or remove the round center insert when blending hot items. The heat will create expansion and pressure inside the blender and could cause the lid to pop off while blending. You can also blend smaller portions to ensure your safety.

FOR RAITA: Roast the cumin seeds with ghee in a small pan on medium heat for a few minutes until the seeds start to smell nutty and turn slightly brown. Remove from heat and spoon seeds into a blender with the yogurt, half of the cucumber, and the dill. Blend on low for 30 seconds, then transfer to a small bowl, mixing gently with the remaining cucumber, black pepper, and salt. To serve, pour a tablespoon of raita on each bowl of soup, then garnish with zucchini strips, sprouts, and ground pumpkin seeds.

add it! For non-cleansing times, add ¼ cup (25 g) finely grated Parmesan cheese to the soup after blending and stir until melted.

tips for your type

BREEZE: Add one extra tablespoon of ghee (14 g) and a pinch of black pepper and ground ginger to the soup.

MOUNTAIN: Add ¼ teaspoon black pepper, ¼ teaspoon ground ginger, and one clove garlic, grated or chopped, to the soup. Add ¼ teaspoon mustard seeds to the raita.

warm slaw

Cold and raw foods should be reserved primarily for a hot season when there is a strong need for cooling the internal environment of the body. If you want to enjoy the flavor and texture of raw vegetables in a cooler season or climate, here is a new twist on traditional coleslaw. The vegetables are grated or finely chopped and then lightly water-sautéed to retain the color, fresh flavor, and texture without the cold. Sunflower oil and avocado replace the heavy mayonnaise sauce of traditional coleslaw with good healthy fats.

YIELD · FOUR 1-CUP (139 G) SERVINGS

1 cup (110 g) finely chopped or grated carrots

1 cup (70 g) finely chopped or grated purple cabbage

1 cup (120 g) finely chopped or grated celery root (celeriac)

1 cup (70 g) finely chopped kale

2 tablespoons (30 ml) water

2 tablespoons (30 ml) sunflower oil

¼ cup (16 g) minced dill

pinch of mineral salt

1 lime, squeezed

1 ripe avocado, sliced

Combine the chopped carrots, cabbage, celery root, and kale in a sauté pan with the water and a splash of sunflower oil. Sauté, covered, on medium heat for 4–7 minutes. A shorter cooking time will retain the firm texture of the vegetables, while a longer time will make them softer and easier to digest. Remove from heat and add the remaining sunflower oil, dill, salt, and lime juice, then mix thoroughly. Add sliced avocado for garnish.

tips for your type

BREEZE: Use sesame oil cooked with a little chopped garlic, add chopped chives, and cook longer.

MOUNTAIN: Use sesame oil cooked with 1 clove garlic, 1 chilli pepper, and chives (all chopped) and cook for a moderate amount of time. Omit avocado.

green beauty sauté

In Ayurvedic consultations, I often tell clients who need a cooling diet to start by eating more green vegetables. This one tip will ensure that they eat more foods with the sweet and bitter tastes that are ideal for reducing heat. Most flower petals also have these two tastes, so any edible varieties are a beautiful complement to green salads or sautés. Many flowers and the essential oils extracted from them are used as remedies to open the heart and to clear heated emotions like anger or frustration. It is easy to be captured by the beauty of a flower and to sink into a moment of stillness in appreciation and awe. One simple way to include more awe-inspiring beauty in your food is by soaking broccoli or broccoli rabe in water and allowing it to blossom.

YIELD · FOUR 1½-CUP (170 G) SERVINGS

2 tablespoons (30 ml) water

1 teaspoon (5 ml) sunflower oil

1 cup (100 g) chopped Romanesco

½ cup (50 g) chopped leek

1 cup (71 g) flowering broccoli rabe

½ cup (35 g) chopped Treviso (bitter green variety of radicchio)

2 cups (135 g) chopped kale, three varieties

20 pea pods (60 g)

20 green beans (100 g)

1 teaspoon (5 ml) rose water or neroli (orange blossom) water, optional

pinch of mineral salt

FOR GARNISH:

sweet pea flowers or other edibles

mint or basil

In a large sauté pan or wok, combine all ingredients. Start with the water and oil, then place harder vegetables like Romanesco, leek, and broccoli rabe in the pan and layer on top the lighter, softer, or leafy vegetables. Cover and cook on medium heat for 5–10 minutes so that the harder vegetables are lightly crunchy and the leafy vegetables start to wilt. Sprinkle the rose or neroli water and salt over the vegetables and then remove from heat. Garnish with edible flowers, mint, or basil and serve.

tips for your type

BREEZE: Include more of the sweeter green vegetables like pea pods and green beans and reduce the amount of strong bitters like Treviso. Cook a few minutes longer to ensure that the harder vegetables are soft, and cook in ghee instead of sunflower oil.

MOUNTAIN: Steam vegetables and sprinkle black pepper on top.

hold the fire please tofu tacos

I love spicy, authentic Mexican food, but it is not always good for my Breezy-Fire constitution. I found a way to enjoy my favorite dishes with less spice, no dairy, and little fat. This recipe is a favorite of my closest friends! It has been growing and changing for two decades, and has now become a Fire-reducing dream come true. You can turn it into a wrap or eat it over a bed of greens as a salad.

YIELD · FOUR LARGE WRAPS OR SIX SMALL WRAPS

1 cup (250 g) black beans, soaked overnight

2 strips of kombu

3 cups (710 g) water

1 teaspoon (3 g) chili powder

1 teaspoon (3 g) ground cumin

salt to taste

1 mango, chopped into ½-inch (13 mm) pieces

½ orange bell pepper, chopped into ½-inch (13 mm) pieces

15 sweet cherry tomatoes (fresh and in season), quartered

¼ cup (4 g) finely chopped cilantro

FOR TOFU STRIPS:
15-ounce (425 g) package of tofu, drained

½ lime, squeezed

¼ teaspoon ground cumin

⅛ teaspoon chili powder

sprinkle or spray liquid aminos

FOR SAUTÉ:
1 cup (95 g) chopped fennel root

1 cup (70 g) chopped baby bok choy

1 cup (80 g) pea pods

½ teaspoon (3 g) ghee

2 tablespoons (30 ml) water

squeeze of lemon or lime

pinch of mineral salt

FOR FRESH TOPPINGS:
¼ cup (28 g) grated carrots

¼ cup (28 g) grated celery root or jicama

1 cup (55 g) chopped lettuce or green cabbage

1 avocado, sliced

whole wheat or sprouted grain tortillas or wraps

Place the black beans in water and soak overnight. Drain the beans, then combine with 3 cups (710 ml) of water and bring to a boil on high heat. Reduce the heat to low and simmer. After one hour, check the beans for tenderness and add the chili powder, cumin, and salt. Continue cooking for 5–30 minutes, until the beans are tender and easily chewed. If the beans start to look dry during the cooking process, add more water ⅛ cup (30 ml) at a time.

Cool the beans and then add mango, bell pepper, cherry tomatoes, and cilantro and stir. Add a splash of olive oil if the beans are dry or sticky.

FOR THE TOFU STRIPS: Drain the water from the tofu, then slice into three ½-inch (13 mm) slabs. Place one clean towel under the tofu on a cutting board or hard surface and another towel over the tofu. Use a large cookbook to press down firmly and evenly on the tofu for 1 minute, then allow it to stay pressed with the weight of the cookbook for another 10 minutes. Slice the tofu into ½-inch (12.5 mm) strips and place in an oven-safe baking dish or on a baking sheet. Squeeze the lime over the tofu strips, then sprinkle the spices and liquid aminos on top to coat the strips evenly. Bake at 375°F (190°C) for 10–15 minutes and flip the pieces over after 8 minutes. *continued on page 184 »*

tofu tacos, continued

FOR THE SAUTÉ: Place all ingredients in a medium sauté pan and water-sauté (see page 114 for details).

Assemble all of the cooked ingredients (black bean salsa, sautéed veggies, and tofu strips) with all of the fresh ingredients (carrots, celery root/jicama, green cabbage/lettuce, and avocado) in a tortilla/wrap or eat over a bed of greens.

tips for your type

BREEZE: Add 1 teaspoon ground ginger and hing to the black beans while cooking. Use yellow onion instead of fennel in the sauté. Use lemon instead of lime on the tofu.

MOUNTAIN: Add 1 teaspoon ginger powder and ½ red onion diced to the black beans while cooking. Substitute a green bell pepper for fennel root in the sauté and a gluten-free tortilla for whole wheat. For the tofu, double the spices and use lemon instead of lime.

BUILDING THE TISSUES

According to Ayurveda, the body is built of seven tissues: *chyle* (plasma), blood, muscle, fat, bone, nervous tissue, and reproductive tissue. The principle "like increases like" applies to foods that are similar to our tissues. For example, fatty foods like avocado and cold-pressed oils help build healthy fat stores and foods abundant in iron, such as molasses, help build blood. When a person is depleted, meat, or the muscle of an animal, is an appropriate food-medicine to build muscle tissue. Likewise, broth made from the marrow of animal bones can also nourish our bone tissue. Vegetarians can use medicinal mushrooms instead. Mushrooms are rather dense, like our muscle tissue, so they too can be nourishing.

grilled summer squash with pesto couscous

If a busy summer schedule keeps you out of the kitchen all day and you return home with a voracious appetite but no dinner, try this. It's easy to prepare, especially if you make the pesto in advance and refrigerate it—and it's ready in just a few minutes.

YIELD · FOUR ½-CUP (79 G) SERVINGS OF COUSCOUS OVER SQUASH AND ZUCCHINI; 1½ CUPS (353 ML) PESTO

1–2 cups (235–475 ml) water

1 cup (175 g) large couscous

1 large zucchini, sliced into large coins

1 large yellow squash, sliced into large coins

1 teaspoon (5 ml) olive oil

FOR PESTO:
¾ cup (102 g) pine nuts

1 cup (40 g) finely chopped basil

1 cup (15 g) cilantro

2 tablespoon (7 g) nutritional yeast

¼ cup (60 ml) olive oil

1 tablespoon (15 ml) water

¼ avocado

½ lemon, squeezed

mineral salt to taste

Place water in a medium saucepan and bring to a boil over high heat. Add couscous, reduce heat to low, and simmer for 5 minutes before pouring off the remaining water. Let stand for a few minutes and fluff with a fork.

Place zucchini and squash in a large bowl and lightly oil before placing on a grill pan or outdoor grill. Cook for a few minutes on medium-high heat to soften the vegetables.

FOR PESTO: Place all ingredients in a blender and puree on high for 1 minute or until creamy.

TO SERVE: Place grilled zucchini and squash on a plate, cover with a scoop of couscous, and pour the pesto over the top.

tips for your type

BREEZE: Add a small clove of garlic to the pesto.

MOUNTAIN: Add 2 cloves of garlic to the pesto and grill the vegetables without oil to dry up moisture. Eat in moderation.

add it! For non-cleansing meals, sprinkle grated Parmesan cheese on top.

hijiki rainbow salad with avocado pumpkin-seed dressing

Seaweed is a nutrient-packed, mineral-rich food that can bring the perfect amount of salt to the Fire's diet. You can choose from many varieties of seaweed; some can be cooked with foods to improve digestion or flavor and others are eaten dried or rehydrated. I cook kombu with beans to improve digestion and reduce gas. Dulse is great dried and chopped into small pieces to sprinkle on salads or soups. Nori is a perfect healthy snack, toasted in the oven with a little oil and rock salt. Hijiki comes dry and needs to be rehydrated before eating, but it can be eaten raw or cooked to add more flavor. This recipe is inspired by a salad I have enjoyed at my favorite sushi restaurant, Bizen, in Western Massachusetts. I have added more sweetness with golden raisins and jicama, a root with the light and crunchy texture of a water chestnut and an apple-like flavor.

YIELD · FOUR TO SIX 1-CUP (200-133 G) SERVINGS DEPENDING ON THE VOLUME OF THE LETTUCE VARIETY

12–16 ounces (340–455 g) of leafy greens, like frisée, green or red leaf lettuce, or baby kale

3 small bell peppers, julienned

¼ small jicama, sliced into matchsticks or grated

1 small carrot, sliced into matchsticks or grated

½ cucumber, peeled and sliced into matchsticks

¼ cup (34 g) golden raisins

¼ cup (6 g) dry hijiki, soaked

1 teaspoon (5 ml) olive oil

squeeze of lemon or lime

sprinkle of maple syrup

FOR DRESSING:

¼ cup (36 g) pumpkin seeds, soaked

⅛ to ¼ cup (30–60 ml) water

1 ripe avocado

1 tablespoon (15 ml) apple cider vinegar

⅛ cup (8 g) chopped parsley, mint, or scallions

1 tablespoon (15 ml) sunflower oil

NOTE: You can aid digestion of raw foods with a small amount of heating foods or spices. The right amount of heat for each person varies, and some Fire individuals will not be able to tolerate any heating foods. Modify as needed to make sure you do not feel any discomfort or heat sensations in the stomach after a meal. In this recipe, the bell peppers are sweet and juicy but have a mild heating nature; apple cider vinegar is sour but used in small amounts; and scallions are heating, parsley slightly less heating, and mint cooling. Choose the mix of ingredients that works for you.

Wash and place leafy salad greens in a large salad serving bowl and arrange chopped vegetables and raisins on top of the greens. Rehydrate hijiki in a bowl of water for 10 minutes, then drain and place in a small sauté pan with oil, lemon or lime, and maple syrup. Cook on low for 15 minutes to tenderize the seaweed and allow the flavors to be absorbed. Place the hijiki in a mound in the center of the greens and serve with dressing.

continued on page 188 »

hijiki salad, *continued*

FOR DRESSING: Soak pumpkin seeds for several hours in a cup of water, then drain and place in a blender with all other ingredients. Blend on low, then on high for a few minutes to make a creamy pourable dressing. More water will make it thinner and easier to spread evenly on the salad.

tips for your type

BREEZE: Raw foods are hard to digest, so use softer, sweeter lettuce varieties and eat only in a warm season. Alternately, eliminate the cucumbers, choose baby kale greens, and lightly sauté all ingredients with the hijiki. Use umeboshi vinegar instead of apple cider vinegar in the dressing.

MOUNTAIN: Eliminate cucumbers, choose baby kale greens, add ½ jalepeño pepper (diced), and lightly sauté all ingredients with the hijiki. For the dressing, add ¼ teaspoon grated ginger and a sprinkle of black pepper and add an extra ¼ cup (60 ml) of water to make it thinner.

quinoa tabouli nori rolls

This dish is fun to prepare and eat. It's an easy finger food to take on the go for a quick meal or snack. Nori, a variety of seaweed, is made into paper-like sheets often used for rolling up sushi. You can find it with other sushi supplies and seaweed varieties in your local co-op or Japanese market.

YIELD · 5-6 NORI ROLLS; SERVING SIZE: ONE TO TWO ROLLS

2 cups (475 ml) water

½ cup (115 g) sushi rice, uncooked

½ cup (86 g) tricolor quinoa, uncooked

¾ cup (45 g) finely chopped parsley

⅛ cup (12 g) finely chopped mint

1 tablespoon (15 ml) olive oil

½ lemon, squeezed

½ lime, squeezed

pinch of mineral salt

FOR NORI ROLLS:
6 sheets of nori

½ avocado, sliced into matchsticks

½ cucumber, peeled and sliced in to matchsticks

Place the water, rice, and quinoa in a rice cooker and press the setting for sushi rice or white rice. Alternately, use a medium saucepan and bring the water to a boil on high heat, add the rice and quinoa, stir, and reduce heat to low. Simmer covered for 15–20 minutes or until the water is absorbed. Remove from heat and let cool for 10–15 minutes. Add parsley, mint, olive oil, lemon, lime, and a pinch of mineral salt (optional) and stir gently to mix ingredients together.

Place a sheet of nori, rough side up, on a flattened bamboo roller, and scoop ½ cup tabouli mix onto the lower third of the sheet. Flatten the mix evenly from side to side and leave a small ½- to 1-inch (13- to 25-mm) line of nori exposed at the bottom. Place a few matchsticks of avocado and cucumber across the tabouli. Moisten the exposed nori with a few drops of water above and below the tabouli and begin rolling. Hold the lower edge of the bamboo against the nori and use it to roll the lower edge over the tabouli. Pull the roller back toward you to tighten the nori periodically as you continue rolling it up.

When the roll is complete, transfer it to a cutting board and use a sharp knife to slice into six or seven ½- to ¾-inch (14 mm) "coins" and serve.

tips for your type

BREEZE: When they are in season, add a few fresh cherry tomatoes, finely chopped, to the tabouli mix.

MOUNTAIN: Eat in moderation with wasabi paste (wasabi powder mixed with a small amount of water). Wasabi powder is made from horseradish, which has a sharp, penetrating heat to aid digestion and will also clear your sinuses.

taking it deeper

—

traditional ayurvedic cleansing

IN THE DAILY PRACTICES OF AYURVEDA, the main goal is pacifying the doshas so that they are not creating problems or imbalances in the body. The excess doshas accumulate over time and at some point pacification is not enough; the doshas need to be removed. Daily and seasonal self-care practices that focus on prevention only pacify the doshas, but when health is lost, Ayurveda recommends an intensive system of cleansing and rejuvenation, called panchakarma, to eliminate excess doshas along with environmental toxins and accumulated ama. For our purposes, this practice is called eliminatory cleansing.

PANCHAKARMA RETREATS

Panchakarma refers to the five (pancha) actions (karmas) used to cleanse accumulated doshas and ama from the body. These five actions are *vamana* (emesis or therapeutic vomiting), *virechana* (purgation from castor oil or herbal formulas), *niruha basti* (herbalized enema, sometimes called cleansing enemas), *nasya* (herbal oils or dry herbs administered through the nostrils), and *anuvasana basti* (oil enema, sometimes called nourishing enemas). Sometimes *rakta moksha*, or mild blood-letting, is named as the fifth action, instead of anu-vasana basti, but that is not as common a practice. It is also not to be compared with the very depleting and excessive use of blood-letting that has historically been used, often to great detriment.

When people discuss the panchakarma process, however, they are usually referring not only to these five cleansing actions but also the preparatory and post-panchakarma stages of a comprehensive cleanse. This comprehensive cleanse includes preparing the body to receive the five actions safely and effectively, undergoing one or more of the five actions, supporting the body to stabilize afterward, and, finally, rejuvenating the body and mind. Traditionally, it is a process that takes a minimum of one month but often several months to complete.

In India, a patient would stay at a hospital or clinic for the entire length of the process and be completely isolated from stressors of life with little or no contact with the outside world. Panchakarma would be completed under the direct supervision of an Ayurvedic doctor, or *vaidya*, and patients would be cared for with daily massage treatments, oils, herbs, food, and rest recommended specifically for their particular imbalance. The ultimate goal of this process was full and complete rejuvenation of all of the bodily tissues, the senses, the mind, and emotions. It was reported to rejuvenate even bone, teeth, and hair of elderly individuals, adding thirty to forty years to their life span.

Although it is still possible to receive this traditional treatment in some places in India, most modern-day panchakarma programs, especially in the West, have been modified to make them more accessible. First, they are designed to allow the client to stay at home for most of the process. This limits the residential time in the personal care of the vaidya. In this way clients can reduce their time away from home and daily life to one or two weeks, making it more accessible to most people. This, however, does make the experience much different and less intense and comprehensive than the traditional system allows. It also places the client in the position of taking personal responsibility for carrying out most of the preparations before and rejuvenation after cleansing without direct supervision.

THE FOUR STAGES OF PANCHAKARMA

The traditional comprehensive cleanse that we usually refer to as panchakarma has four stages. *Ama-pachana*, the first stage, involves practices to burn up ama in the digestive tract, remove congestion and blockages in the channels, and strengthen the digestive fire.

Traditionally, recommended practices would include warm oil massage treatments, very gentle yoga postures or breathing practices to increase the strength of the digestive fire, a simple diet with little to no oil or salt, and herbal teas or medicinal formulas that are pungent, bitter, or astringent in nature. In nonresidential preparations, recommendations usually involve dietary changes, daily cleansing practices, and herbal intake. These practices serve to clear the digestive tract before the second stage, so that the ingested ghee does not create more congestion.

Stage two aims to lubricate the digestive tract and soften the tissues. This is accomplished internally with ingestion of ghee and externally with the application of oil and heat. Oleation, or application of oil (*snehana*, see sidebar on right), and sudation, application of heat (*swedana*), are the two main therapies used to move the accumulated doshas from their locations around the body back to their homesites. The purpose of this stage is to soften the tissues, open subtle channels of the body, and create a clear pathway for old stored toxins and accumulated doshas to return to the digestive tract for elimination from the body through the five actions. The cleansing actions to remove the excess doshas cannot be carried out safely unless the oleation process is done properly. The goal is to saturate the tissues thoroughly from the inside and the outside.

In the third stage, each of the five actions of panchakarma is used to remove one or more of the accumulated doshas. Not all clients need all of the actions. Some clients may need only one action, while others may need several. *Bastis*, or enemas, remove excess vata dosha. Purgation with castor oil or other herbal formulas removes excess pitta dosha. Therapeutic vomiting, or vamana, removes excess kapha dosha. Mild blood-letting, or rakta moksha, removes excess pitta, and nasya, or therapies applied through the nostrils, removes accumulated doshas from the brain, nervous system, or the mind. Even today, blood-letting is often performed with leeches for obstinate skin diseases or stubborn, chronic, localized pain. The leeches are usually applied near the area of the skin eruption or the area of pain, to draw fresh blood through the problem area. Rakta moksha is rarely practiced in the West, though some vaidyas may recommend that certain individuals with high pitta donate blood.

The deepest part of the cleansing process is carried out during the third stage, but the cleansing does not stop there. In fact, the actions of panchakarma really just open the flood gates, so that the body can continue the cleansing process for the next few months. It is very important to understand that this final phase of rejuvenation is just as important as any other stage.

The body is in a vulnerable state at this point in the process, because the excess doshas that were eliminated may have been accumulating for decades and the body has compensated for these imbalances. Imagine pulling a weed up out of the ground and observing the space in the soil the roots occupied. This empty space in the soil is much like the empty space in the body after the excess doshas have been removed. It takes time and proper care to rebuild healthy, strong, balanced tissues to fill the weak spaces. Rejuvenation, the fourth stage, takes one to three months to complete. Ayurvedic doctors often recommend that patients care for themselves during this period as if they have just had surgery.

The rejuvenation period consists of daily self-care practices, diet, herbal preparations, and lifestyle recommendations tailored to each individual to rebuild healthy tissues and prevent future accumulation of the imbalanced doshas. The diet only gradually becomes heavier and more

OLEATION

Picture a twig on a tree—it is soft, green, flexible, and full of sap. It does not break easily. This is the state of our human bodies as children—soft, juicy, and flexible. Like a twig that has fallen off the tree, we become drier and more brittle with age. Now imagine taking that dry twig, soaking it in warm oil, and steaming it. The oil will penetrate into the small channels or openings and saturate it. Eventually, the twig will be flexible enough to bend and twist again without breaking. This is the goal of oleation in panchakarma.

nourishing than during the cleansing process, and herbal formulas are often sweet and building in nature. Daily oil massage with specific oils is recommended, as well as the daily routine of cleansing practices for the organs of elimination and the senses (dinacharya). Yoga, breathing practices, exercise, and rest are prescribed in proper amounts for rejuvenation.

THE GHEE CLEANSE

When panchakarma is not possible—due to time constraints, finances, or other factors—but a deeper cleanse is required, some Ayurvedic practitioners will suggest a ghee cleanse. These individually tailored practices take several forms, but the common link is using ghee to cleanse (similar to the second phase of panchakarma). Just as in panchakarma, this practice requires guidance by a professional. Some practitioners call it a "home panchakarma," as Dr. Vasant Lad describes in the book *Ayurvedic Home Remedies*, while other practitioners incorporate it with other cleansing practices, as Dr. John Douillard does in his book *Colorado Cleanse*. These are modern adaptations not mentioned in the classic texts.

Ghee cleanses typically involve burning up ama and toxins in the digestive tract, and this is accomplished through eating a lightening diet similar to the final days of your month-long protocol and taking pungent, bitter, or astringent herbs and teas. Then ghee is ingested in increasing amounts for a period of four to seven days, during which kitchari is the recommended mono diet. A daily self-massage with warm oils is followed by application of heat for all or some of the cleansing days.

After the oleation is complete, castor oil or other purgatives are administered to release the contents of the digestive tract and eliminate the excess doshas that have returned to their homesites from the process of oleation. One or more days of rest is recommended for rejuvenation, along with an oil enema to nourish and soothe the colon.

WHY CLEANSE WITH GHEE?

Ayurveda considers ghee the best food-medicine. It lubricates the mucosae of the digestive tract, helps regulate digestion and hormones, lubricates the joints, and can increase good cholesterol. It can penetrate into minute channels of the body, opening and clearing them to restore proper flow of oxygen, nutrients, and waste products.

Our guiding intelligence will store toxins or impurities away from the circulation and flow of daily metabolic activities. The storage site of choice is our adipose tissue, or fat. Even on a cellular level, toxins are stored in and transported by fat molecules. The cell membrane is permeable by fat, so it makes sense that to cleanse the body of unwanted wastes, a lipophilic, or fat-loving, substance would be the ideal carrier. Ghee is that ideal carrier.

The ghee cleanse is appropriate for those who have adequate strength to undergo the purgation process, because, like panchakarma, it not only removes ama and toxins (as many modern cleanses do), but also goes a step further to remove the excess doshas. This is a deeper cleanse and requires more strength to complete without creating imbalance.

PARTNERING WITH AN AYURVEDIC PROFESSIONAL

It is a goal of Ayurveda to empower individuals to take responsibility for their own health and use the tools of self-awareness and practices of self-care to create balance. Still, it is also a good idea to have an experienced guide along the way, particularly in cases when imbalance has already progressed through the six stages to a fully manifested disease.

Improper practices of cleansing can drive the doshas and toxins deeper into the body and create more imbalance. Only experienced Ayurvedic doctors are qualified to advise patients on the state of health for maintenance and the state of disease. They can navigate the challenging and complicated world of allopathic medicine and pharmaceutical drugs and weave its approaches masterfully with the herbal remedies and natural practices of Ayurveda. For deep cleansing, this guidance is essential: Panchakarma should never be done without an Ayurvedic doctor or an experienced practitioner.

An Ayurvedic practitioner or lifestyle consultant who is not trained specifically in panchakarma practices can still advise about practices for maintaining health and balancing the doshas when they have become aggravated. An Ayurvedic professional can recommend food-medicines and spices as well as daily self-care practices, yoga poses, breathing practices, lifestyle changes, Ayurvedic

bodywork therapies, and daily, dietary, or digestive cleansing practices. Truly, the simple basics of Ayurveda are so powerful when practiced regularly that these can often bring about life-changing improvements.

CONSTITUTION CHECKLIST

— courtesy of banyan botanicals,
created by dr. claudia welch —

Place a check mark next to each statement that has applied to you throughout your life. Total the number of checks in each category to determine your predominance.

_ My lifelong tendency has been to be thin and lanky.

_ I find having a routine in life challenging.

_ My skin tends to be rough and dry, even if I don't live in a dry, arid climate (and especially if I do).

_ My joints are fairly prominent.

_ My teeth are protruded and/or crooked.

_ My hair is kinky, curly, and tends to be dry or frizzy.

_ It is usually easy for me to lose weight and I usually have difficulty gaining weight.

_ I usually enjoy hot weather.

_ I tend to dislike wind.

_ I tend to dislike very dry climates.

Total Breeze/vata characteristics: _____

_ I have a medium build with medium bone structure.

_ I enjoy competitive activities and enjoy physical or intellectual challenges.

_ My teeth are medium-sized and/or a little yellow (stained doesn't count).

_ I have fair skin that sunburns easily.

_ I have a lot of moles or freckles.

_ I am or am becoming bald, I have grayed early, or I have thin or fine hair.

_ My eyes are sensitive to light.

_ I prefer a cool climate to a warm one.

_ I dislike heat, especially humid heat, and feel easily fatigued by it.

_ I have a sharp, intelligent, aggressive mind.

Total Fire/pitta characteristics: _____

_ I have a sturdy constitution with a large bone structure.

_ I have had a lifelong tendency to always be at least a little overweight.

_ My teeth are naturally large, straight, and white.

_ My hair is thick and lustrous.

_ My eyes are large with long, full, luxurious lashes.

_ If given the opportunity, I can easily sleep deeply for 8–10 hours per night.

_ I gain weight easily and have difficulty losing weight.

_ My facial features are rounded, with full, moist lips.

_ I tolerate most climates well, but have usually preferred hot, dry weather.

_ My energy and stamina are consistent. When I have a lot to do, I do it at a pace that I can maintain for a long time.

Total Mountain/kapha characteristics: _____

IMBALANCE
CHECKLIST

— courtesy of banyan botanicals,
created by dr. claudia welch —

Place a check mark next to each statement that applies to you at this time. Total the number of checks in each category to find your predominant imbalance.

_ I have been feeling nervous, fearful, panicky, anxious, or frantic.

_ I have twitches, tics, tremors, or spasms in my body and I fidget a lot.

_ My skin is dry and easily chapped.

_ I have been suffering from dry, hard stools, constipation, gas, or bloating, or I have been having loose stools due to emotional upset.

_ I feel I am underweight.

_ Lately I have a stronger dislike of the wind and cold than usual.

_ I have a difficult time tolerating loud noise.

_ My sleep has been light, interrupted, restless, or disturbed.

_ I feel scattered, spacey, and have difficulty concentrating or have poor memory.

_ I am prone to overthinking or worrying.

Total Breeze/vata imbalances: _____

_ I have a red, inflamed, or burning rash; acne, cold sores, or fever blisters.

_ There is acute inflammation in my body or joints.

_ I have acid reflux, heartburn, acid indigestion, or a gastric or peptic ulcer—or a tight, burning feeling in my stomach or digestive tract.

_ I feel nauseated or uncomfortable if I miss a meal.

_ I have been having loose stools that are not due to emotional upset.

_ I have been feeling uncomfortably warm or hot.

_ I have been feeling frustrated, irritable, or angry.

_ I can be easily judgmental, impatient, critical, or intolerant of others.

_ My eyes have been red, bloodshot, inflamed, or sensitive to light.

_ I expect perfection of myself or others.

Total Fire/pitta imbalances: _____

_ I have excess mucus in my body or nasal passages or lung congestion.

_ I have a thick, white coating on my tongue.

_ My bowel movements are slow, sticky, sluggish, or feel incomplete.

_ I am overweight.

_ It is difficult for me to wake up in the mornings, even if I sleep deeply for 8–10 hours, and I feel lethargic throughout the day.

_ I have been feeling slow, foggy, dull, lethargic, or heavy.

_ In the morning I have to cough up a lot of mucus.

_ I have a deep, wet cough that produces a lot of mucus.

_ I feel complacent, stubborn, and resistant to any change—or my close friends and family tell me that I am very slow to change or to make a decision.

_ I am prone to excessive emotional eating, especially of sweet, heavy foods.

Total Mountain/kapha imbalances: _____

cleansing table

When picking a cleanse, you should choose one to correct your predominant imbalance. If, after taking the Constitution and Imbalance Questionnaires, you have more than one predominant imbalance, refer to the table below to determine which cleanse is right for you. If you are balanced, then you should pick your cleanse based your constitution, with mindful consideration of the season.

USING THE TABLE

Step 1 Find your constitution in the far left column.
Step 2 Move across the chart to find your predominant imbalances and use the key below to determine which cleanse is appropriate (G, C, or L) and if you need modifications (*b, *f, *m, in cold, in hot, or in particular seasons).
Possible Imbalances:

BF: equally predominant Breeze and Fire imbalances
BM: equally predominant Breeze and Mountain imbalances
FM: equally predominant Fire and Mountain imbalances
BFM: Breeze, Fire, and Mountain imbalances equally

Key to Cleanse Options:
G: Grounding
C: Cooling
L: Lightening

Key to Modification Options:
  ÷ *b: Use the Breeze modifications.
  ÷ *f: Use the Fire modifications.
  ÷ *m: Use the Mountain modifications.
  ÷ in cold: Use in a cold or cool season.
  ÷ in hot: Use in a hot or warm season.

cleansing table

CONSTITUTION	IDEAL SEASON	BF IMBALANCES	BM IMBALANCES	FM IMBALANCES	BFM IMBALANCES
BREEZE	Autumn	G in cold/C in hot	G or L*b	C in hot/ L in cold	G
BREEZE-FIRE	Between summer/autumn	G in cold/ C in hot	G or L*b	C in hot/ L in cold	G
BREEZE-MOUNTAIN	Autumn + spring	G in cold/ C in hot	G in autumn/ L*b in summer/ L in spring	C in hot/ L in cold	G or L*b
FIRE	Beginning and end of summer	G in cold/ C in hot	G in autumn/ L other times	C in hot/ L*f in cold	C
FIRE-BREEZE	Between summer/autumn	G in cold/ C in hot	G in autumn/ G*m in summer/ L in spring	C in hot/ L*f in cold	C in hot/ G in cold
FIRE-MOUNTAIN	Between spring/ summer	G in cold/ C in hot	G in autumn/ L other times	C*m in hot/ L*f in cold	C in hot/ L*f other
MOUNTAIN	Early spring	G in cold/ C in hot	G in autumn/ L other times	C in hot/ L other	L
MOUNTAIN-BREEZE	Spring + autumn	G in cold/ C in hot	G*m or L	C in hot/ L other	L or L*b
MOUNTAIN-FIRE	Between spring/ summer	G in cold/ C in hot	G*m or L	C*m in hot/ L*f in cold	L*f in cold/ C*m in hot
BREEZE-FIRE-MOUNTAIN	Between spring/ summer + summer/autumn	G in cold/ C in hot	G autumn/ L other	C in hot/ L in cold	G autumn/ C summer/ L spring

the five elements

The five elements are the basic substances or building blocks of the universe and the body. We are each composed of all five elements, and the doshas of Vata (Breeze), Pitta (Fire), and Kapha (Mountain) are also made up of them. However, each dosha has a predominance of certain qualities related to two of the five elements.

Ether is the space of the universe—our planet, our homes, and our bodies all occupy a space and have spaces within them. Ether is light, clear, expansive, and subtle. In the body, it exists in the spaces of the lungs, the hollow tube-like space of the colon, the spaces in the porous structure of the bones, and the space inside each cell.

Air is movement through a space. This element is present in all movement. It is mobile, dry, light, subtle, cold, and rough. In the body, air relates to the pulsation of the heart, the movement of the lungs, and all stimuli that move through the nervous system.

The qualities of **ether** and **air** predominate in **vata** dosha.

Fire is the heat of transformation: Movement creates friction, friction creates heat, and heat creates the fire that carries out transformation. It is hot, sharp, light, dry, and subtle. In the body, the transformation of digestion, body temperature, and metabolic transformation inside each cell are examples of fire.

Water is the liquid element that allows cohesion, nourishment, and cleansing. It is cool, moist, dull, and soft. In the body, it relates to the lubricating liquid in the joints and the plasma content of blood. Plasma, which is 90 percent water, is the fluid that carries all nutrients and oxygen to the cells for nourishment and all of the waste products away for cleansing.

The qualities of **fire** and **water** predominate in **pitta** dosha.

Earth is the dense, hard element that composes all solid structures. It is heavy, stable, dull, and gross. In the body, it is the firm, hard, and compact tissues such as the bones, nails, teeth, and hair.

The qualities of **water** and **earth** predominate in the **kapha** dosha.

AYURVEDIC BODYWORK GUIDE
— *courtesy of lakshmi's garden* —

Abhyanga: A powerfully relaxing, warm-oil massage with gentle to firm pressure and long fluid strokes to calm the body and mind

Good for: insomnia, anxiety, restlessness, stress, overwork, dryness, and exhaustion

Benefits: calms nervous system; increases lymphatic flow to aid detoxification; improves circulation; rejuvenates; and balances Vata dosha (Breeze)

Garshana: An invigorating dry massage with raw silk gloves that stimulates the body's healing energies and prepares the skin to absorb herbalized oils

Good for: dry skin, sluggishness, and lethargy

Benefits: exfoliates and rejuvenates skin; increases circulation of blood and lymphatic flow; aids in detoxification; energizes, uplifts, and balances all doshas—used in moderation for Vata dosha (Breeze)

Kati Basti: A mold of flours shaped around the low back and sacrum that creates a reservoir for warm oil

Good for: low back tension or pain; stiff or sore muscles; conditions of the lumbar spine; sciatica; urinary, excretory, or reproductive system imbalances; and constipation

Benefits: relaxes muscles of the low back, sacrum, and pelvic region (softens and warms tissues and opens the channels) to restore balance; calms the nervous system; rejuvenates the spinal column; and balances Vata dosha (Breeze)

Marma: Gentle stimulation of the 108 energy centers of the body by means of touch therapy and aromatherapy that rebalances the pranic body and creates an overall sense of peace and well-being

Good for: conditions of the nervous system; chronic tension areas, trauma, or injury; overactive mind; imbalances of prana; and emotional disturbances

Benefits: balances the flow of prana; removes energetic blockages; calms the body, mind, and emotions; stimulates the body's natural healing energy; good for all doshas

Netra Basti: A reservoir is created around the eyes with dough, then the eyes are bathed in ghee or herbal oils

Good for: eyes strain, vision problems, pain or inflammation of the eyes, tension of the face or head, chronic headaches, dry eyes, dry, wrinkled skin around eyes

Benefits: releases inner tension of the eye sockets, soothes dry or heated eyes, improves eyesight, nourishes the central nervous system, reduces Pitta and Vata dosha (Fire and Breeze), calms prana vayu

Potli: Warm bundles of an herbal mixture soaked and heated in medicated oils, then used to massage the body, especially the joints and spine

Good for: muscular aches and pains around joints or spine; imbalances of the spine; joint inflammation; and stiff joints

Benefits: reduces inflammation of the tissues; warms muscles, increasing circulation and relieving tension; rejuvenates joints and spine; and releases adhesions; good for all doshas

Shiro-Abhyanga-Nasya (SAN): A vigorous massage of the head, neck, and shoulders followed by a eucalyptus steam and ginger *nasya* (nasal) drops to clear out congestion of the sinuses and the lymphatics of the upper body

Good for: sinus and lung congestion; allergies; cloudy mind and senses; cough; colds; neck and shoulder tension; and headaches

Benefits: clears sinus congestion; opens breathing passages; aids in draining excess lymph; relaxes muscles; improves mental clarity and sense perception; and balances Kapha dosha (Mountain)

Shirodhara: A stream of warm oil poured over the third-eye area and forehead that works directly on the central nervous system to quiet the mind and deeply relax the entire body

Good for: conditions of the nervous system; anxiety;

insomnia; nervous conditions; headaches; stress; overwork; exhaustion; jaw pain; and restless body and mind

Benefits: relaxes muscles of the head, neck, and shoulders; calms the central nervous system; quiets the mind; may induce profound relaxation and deep states of meditation and balances Vata dosha (Breeze)

Swedna: An herbalized full-body steam to cleanse excess heat and toxins from the tissues, performed on the massage table with a specialized tent; can stand alone or follow any of the bodywork treatments

Good for: heaviness; sluggishness; congestion; muscle aches; joint stiffness; certain skin conditions; and heat intolerance

Benefits: drains the lymphatic system for detoxification; cleanses the body and mind; revitalizes skin; relaxes muscles; and balances all doshas

Udvartina: A stimulating massage with herbal powders and warm oils to powerfully exfoliate and deeply detoxify the tissues

Good for: obesity; lymphatic congestion; sluggishness; detoxification or cleansing; and certain skin conditions

Benefits: cleanses and nourishes the skin; increases circulation and lymphatic flow; breaks down excess adipose tissue; and reduces Kapha dosha (Mountain)

Vishesh: A vigorous, rhythmic massage with warm oil and firm, deep pressure to remove adhesions in the muscle and connective tissue

Good for: muscle aches and pains; mental tension; stiff joints; and sluggishness

Benefits: relaxes the body and mind; releases adhesions in muscle and connective tissue; improves circulation, joint mobility, and lymphatic flow; warms the tissues; and balances Kapha and Pitta doshas (Mountain and Fire)

resources

AYURVEDIC SUPPLIES:

www.banyanbotanicals.com
Base oils, doshic oils, herbs (including ananta mula, Indian chocolate), mung beans, Ayurvedic supplies, and books

www.saradausa.com
Traditional Ayurvedic doshic oils and skin care

www.osiliving.com
Nontraditional Ayurvedic oils and body products

www.ayurveda.com
Wide variety of Ayurvedic supplies, including audio and video, books, body care, foods, herbs, and specialty oils

GARSHANA (RAW SILK) GLOVES:

www.lakshmisgarden.com
Adjustable drawstring gloves with Velcro closures

www.lifespa.com
Gloves with snap closures

www.ajaraskincare.com
Pull-on gloves

PANCHAKARMA IN THE UNITED STATES:

Lakshmi's Garden in Western Massachusetts
www.lakshmisgarden.com

The Ayurvedic Institute in Albuquerque, New Mexico
www.ayurveda.com

The Ayurvedic Center of Vermont
www.ayurvedavermont.com

The Raj in Fairfield, Iowa
www.theraj.com

LifeSpa in Boulder, Colorado
www.lifespa.com

PANCHAKARMA IN INDIA:

Vaidyagrama near Coimbatore, Tamilnadu
www.vaidyagrama.com

Vinayak Ayurveda and Panchakarma Research Center in Nagpur, Maharashtra
vinayakayurveda.com

Jiva Ayurveda in Faridabad, Haryana
www.jiva.com

VIDEO DEMONSTRATIONS:

Go to www.lakshmisgarden.com for links to videos about using a neti pot, staying in balance, stretching, and more.

bibliography

Buettner, Dan. *The Blue Zones: Lessons for Living Longer from the People Who've Lived the Longest.* Washington, D.C.: National Geographic, 2008.

Dash, Vaidya Bhagwan, and Ram Karan Sharma. *Charaka Samhita.* Delhi, India: Nag Publishers, 1995.

Douillard, John. *Colorado Cleanse: 2 Week Detox and Digestion Boot Camp.* United States of America: Lifespa, 2011.

Frawley David. *American Institute of Vedic Studies Ayurvedic Healing Correspondence Course for Health Care Professionals.* Santa Fe, New Mexico: American Institute of Vedic Studies, 1988.

Frawley, Dr. David, and Dr. Vasant Lad. *The Yoga of Herbs: An Ayurvedic Guide to Herbal Medicine.* Twin Lakes, Wisconsin: Lotus Press, 1986.

Frawley, Dr. David, and Sandra Somerfield Kozak. *Yoga for Your Type: An Ayurvedic Approach to Your Asana Practice.* Twin Lakes, Wisconsin: Lotus Press, 2001.

Lad, Vasant. *Textbook of Ayurveda: Fundamental Principles.* Albuquerque, New Mexico: The Ayurvedic Press, 2002.

Lad, Vasant. *Ayurveda: The Science of Self-Healing: A Practical Guide.* Twin Lakes, Wisconsin: Lotus Press, 1985.

Lad, Vasant. *The Complete Book of Ayurvedic Home Remedies.* New York: Three Rivers Press, 1999.

Vagbhata. *Ashtanga Hridayam.* Translated by Prof. K. R. Srikantha Murthy. Varanasi, India: Krishnadas Academy, 2001.

Wolverton, B. C. *How to Grow Fresh Air: 50 Houseplants that Purify Your Home or Office.* New York: Penguin Books, 1997.

WEBSITES AND E-MEDIA

Cottis, Halle. "How-to Video: Making Organic, Pure Stevia and Liquid Stevia." (October 10, 2011). www.wholelifestylenutrition.com. Retrieved from www.wholelifestylenutrition.com/videos/making-pure-stevia-and-liquid-stevia.

Douiilard, Dr. John. "The Truth About Oil Pulling." www.Lifespa.com. (2013, August 1). www.lifespa.com/the-truth-about-oil-pulling.

Hyman, Dr. Mark. (2012, June 19). "If We Can't Cure the Patient, Can the Community Do It?" [Video file]. Retrieved from www.youtube.com/watch?v=8dYTa6xhHlM.

"Mung Bean (Vigna Radiata)." www.feedipedia.org. Retrieved from www.feedipedia.org/node/235.

about the author

Kimberly Larson has over twenty years of experience as a certified massage therapist, yoga teacher, and Ayurvedic consultant. She is a passionate health educator and the co-owner of Lakshmi's Garden, where she offers personalized cleansing and rejuvenating retreats; panchakarma; and private bodywork, yoga, and consultation sessions. Kimberly is a graduate of the Kripalu Schools of Yoga and Ayurveda, is a former Kripalu faculty member, and has completed advanced studies in India and Thailand. She has devoted the past decade to creating personalized health plans for individuals, including daily diet and recipes, personalized yoga and self-care, and tailored cleansing practices. She and her husband Terrel travel nationally and internationally, teaching and spreading their love of Ayurveda.

acknowledgments

Heartfelt thanks to the Allen/Gunderson family for making your home our home (and letting us make it quite a mess!). Thanks to Jean, Deb, Kevin, Lyn, Jo, Naomi, Jolie, and Perry for helping me have space to create; to Lorimer Burns for you generous donation of beautiful pottery; and to Mandala Yoga and Ayurveda Center for yoga wear. Sending gratitude to all my teachers of yoga, massage, and Ayurveda for this enduring knowledge, with special thanks to Dr. Rosy. Love and unending appreciation to Michelle (for everything); and to my dearest teachers, Terrel and Nilani—thank you for all of your support, love, and sacrifice.

INDEX

A

Abhyanga, described, 201

Aging, 16–17

Ama
- creation and effects of, 53–54
- reading tongue coating, 54–56

Ayurveda
- basic information about, 12
- definition of health, 17–18
- goal of longevity, 16–17
- observation walk, 19
- partnering with professional, 195
- principle of like increases like, 34, 184
- principle of opposites, 18, 19, 34
- toolbox of observation, understanding, and transformation, 17

Ayurvedic Home Remedies (Lad), 194

B

Balance
- finding, 19
- *See also* Imbalance

Bed yoga, 70

Blue Zones: 9 Lessons for Living Longer from the People Who've Lived the Longest (Buettner), 16–17

The body
- as house, 29
- intelligence of, 16
- layers, 41, 184
- signals from, 11–12
- twenty qualities in, 18
- *See also* "Food body"

Body-mind types
- Constitution Checklist to determine, 196–197
- overview of, 21–22

Bodywork guide, 201–202

Brahmana (building) category of food, 54

Breakfast porridge and konji, 81

Breathing practices
- cooling cleanse, 160
- grounding cleanse, 97
- lightening cleanse, 129

Breeze body type. *See* Vata/Breeze dosha (body type)

Breeze Checklist, 197–198

Buettner, Dan, 16–17

C

Calming foods, 67

Change of season fasts, 7

Chutney, 85

Cinnamon, 38–39

Cleanses
- background fundamentals necessary for, 9
- categories of, 59–60
- fasts during seasonal transitions, 7
- public, 56
- purpose of, 9
- 31-day, 65–70, 71
- transition time after, 70–71
- during winter, 58
- *See also* Recipes for staple foods for cleanses; specific cleanses and recipes for specific cleanses

Cleansing table, 198–199

Coffee, 168

Colorado Cleanse (Douillard), 194

Constitution, defined, 26

Constitution Checklist, 196–197

Cooking tips
- energizing food, 76–77
- leftovers, 77
- six tastes in each meal, 76
- using rice cookers, 73–75
- weekly preparations, 76

Cooling cleanse and diet
- about, 159
- daily schedule, 162
- daily self-care practices, 159–161
- "eat more" list of foods for, 101, 163

Cooling cleanse and diet recipes
- about, 163
- coconut almond porridge with baked pears and apples, 170
- cool as a cucumber summer cleanse juice, 167
- the cool-down "iced" tea, 165
- creamy cauliflower and wild rice soup, 171
- green beauty sauté, 181
- grilled summer squash with pesto couscous, 185
- hijiki rainbow salad with avocado pumpkin-seed dressing, 187–188

hold the fire please tofu tacos, 183–184

quinoa tabouli nori rolls, 189

summer soothe tea, 166

summer sunrise pudding, 175

"swami's secret" tofu scramble, 172–173

sweet green goodness soup with cucumber raita, 176–177

turmeric "latte," 168–169

warm slaw, 179

D

Daily cleansings, 59

Dietary cleansings, 59

Digestive cleansings, 59–60

Digestive fire
- described, 25
- imbalance and, 28, 29, 48
- importance of balanced, 53
- Kapha/Mountain, 37
- peak of daily, 49
- Pitta/Fire, 38, 39
- tips for balanced, 45–47
- Vata/Breeze, 36
- water temperature, 44

Digestive naps, 88

Disease, six stages of, 55–56

Dosha, translation of, 26–27

Dulling foods, 67–68

E

Eliminatory cleansings, 60–61

Energetics of food, 67–68

Exercise
- cooling cleanse, 160–161
- lightening cleanse, 129

F

Fasts during seasonal transitions, 7

Fire body type. *See* Pitta/Fire dosha (body type)

Five elements, 22, 200

Food
- basics for nourishing "food body," 42–43
- categories of, 54
- cinnamon, 38–39
- coffee, 168

Quarto is the authority on a wide range of topics.

Quarto educates, entertains and enriches the lives of our readers—enthusiasts and lovers of hands-on living.

www.quartoknows.com

First published in the United States of America in 2017 by
Fair Winds Press, an imprint of
Quarto Publishing Group USA Inc.
100 Cummings Center
Suite 406-L
Beverly, Massachusetts 01915-6101
Telephone: (978) 282-9590
Fax: (978) 283-2742
QuartoKnows.com
Visit our blogs at QuartoKnows.com

21 20 19 18 17   1 2 3 4 5

ISBN: 978-1-59233-749-1

Library of Congress Cataloging-in-Publication Data available

Design and Page Layout: Stacy Wakefield Forte
Photography: Michelle Allen Photography//www.michellempls.com

Printed in China

The information in this book is for educational purposes only. It is not intended to replace the advice of a physician or medical practitioner. Please see your health-care provider before beginning any new health program.